Department of Social and Administrative Studies,
Barnett House,
Wellington Square,
Oxford.

HOSPITAL CLOSURE

HOSPITAL CLOSURE
A political and economic study

**NANCY KORMAN and
HOWARD GLENNERSTER**

OPEN UNIVERSITY PRESS
Milton Keynes · Philadelphia

Open University Press
12 Cofferidge Close
Stony Stratford
Milton Keynes MK11 1BY

and
1900 Frost Road, Suite 101
Bristol, PA 19007, USA

First Published 1990

British Library Cataloguing in Publication Data
Korman, Nancy
   Hospital closure: a political and economic study.
   1. England. Mental handicap hospitals. Closure
   I. Title   II. Glennerster, Howard
   362.3'85

   ISBN 0–335–15434–4
          0–335–15429–8 (paper)

Library of Congress Cataloging in Publication Number available

Typeset by Scarborough Typesetting Services
Printed in Great Britain by Biddles Ltd
Guildford and King's Lynn

Contents

List of tables

List of figures

Introduction

The Darenth Park Project was the earliest attempt by a Regional Health Authority (RHA) to bring about the complete closure of a large mental handicap hospital which had traditionally served almost half of one Thames Region. The stimulus to this project originally came from an external source – the proposed purchase of the hospital land by Blue Circle Industries Ltd. When this was turned down by a planning enquiry in 1979, the RHA decided to pursue the objective of hospital closure, meeting capital and revenue requirements of new locally based services from within its own resources.

The research project on which this book is based was commissioned by the Mental Handicap Research Liaison Group of the then DHSS, at the request of the Darenth Park Steering Group. NHS and departmental officers saw the hospital closure and transfer of services to locally based units as a unique opportunity to learn from this pioneering activity. The increasing number of authorities which have recently begun to express their intentions to work towards the closure of large mental illness or mental handicap institutions has added to the timeliness of the research.

This study is concerned with the administrative, financial and political issues involved in the closure. Dr Lorna Wing of the MRC Social Psychiatry Research Unit is evaluating the effect the change is having on the residents when they move and their adjustment to new environments. Her work is continuing, but the first results have been published (Wing, 1989). We have drawn on her results and some of her data at various points.

The first stages of this long process of closure were described in an interim report (Korman and Glennerster, 1985). As it turned out, that report was only able to review a long and frustrating period of planning, much of which proved abortive. New approaches to care and financial freedom of action had begun to change the situation just prior to the publication of that report. In the subsequent four years, events moved rapidly and the hospital closed in August 1988. This study covers not only the first period, but also, in more detail, the later more eventful period. It sets the entire closure programme in the context of theoretical debates about 'deinstitutionalization' and 'normalization'. It analyses the national policy and financial context in which closure occurred and the way it affected the outcome. Part 2 is a study of the professional and bureaucratic politics of closure, and Part 3 seeks to describe the outcome for the residents and the economic cost of reproviding services in the community.

Methodology

The primary aim of the research was to present an account of the activities leading to the closure of the hospital as seen by those involved. In order to achieve this it is important not to begin with rigid ideas about the course of events and precise sequence of research activities. We have found it necessary to be open to respond to unexpected events, changing personnel and procedures. Issues emerged during the research which were impossible to foresee at the outset. The importance of the issues can only be defined by the way they are taken up by the participants.

We have elsewhere described our approach as 'administrative anthropology' (Glennerster *et al.*, 1983). By this we mean the use of a variety of sources of information by participants. We have used committee papers, reports and official files to produce abstracts relating to the Darenth project and mental handicap policy in general. Working in the office of the various authorities has provided many opportunities for informal conversations which often reveal more than does a formal interview.

Specifically, at the regional level, we reviewed all of the papers of the Darenth Park Steering Group from the time it was established in 1978, the minutes and relevant papers of meetings of the Regional Health Authority (RHA), the Regional Team of Officers (RTO), the Regional Planning Group (RPG), and the Regional Strategies' Subgroup on Mental Handicap Services, and all of the regional-led project planning teams for district replacement facilities. Files on capital projects pre-dating the Darenth project were consulted – Grove Park (five volumes) and Archery House. And from the Regional Medical Officer's divisions, the files on the Hospital Advisory Service (HAS) visits to Darenth Park and the Regional Advisory Team report on Darenth were examined.

Within the districts, minutes and papers from Health Care Planning Teams or District Planning Teams for Mental Handicap Services were read, as well as AHA and DHA minutes, Joint Care Planning Team and Joint Consultative Committee minutes. Files on local mental handicap provision were also studied.

Similarly, within local authorities, minutes and papers from social services committees and departmental planning groups were consulted and in some cases files on local facilities for mentally handicapped people.

The reports we produced were fed back to key participants and formed the basis of interviews. This allowed officers to correct, amend and enlarge upon the account so that an agreed version resulted. This method also allowed officers to know what the researchers were thinking so that the paper produced became a collaborative understanding of events.

We were also given permission to attend a variety of planning meetings in the various authorities which have been useful for getting to know participants, catch up on what was happening, and get some sense of the 'feel' of the project.

Drafts of our report have been given to participants in each authority for comments and this too has helped to expand and confirm our understanding of the events discussed in the report.

Acknowledgements

Our research was pursued over seven and a half years. During this time, we have acquired many debts of gratitude to officers in health and local authorities, and to staff at all levels in Darenth Park Hospital, for the time they have given to the project. They have given permission to attend meetings, provided access to files, made time available for discussion and generally showed a considerable interest in the research, over a long period of time.

We are also grateful to David Pamment, the Mental Health Planning Co-ordinator, who did so much to keep us informed of how planning issues were being discussed and handled, making us aware of the various constraints being experienced and speedily reading and constructively commenting upon our written material. A special thanks as well to Jeanette Smith who chaired the region's project teams with districts and always made certain we knew of events between meetings.

We wish to record our appreciation to the direct care staff and residents who allowed us to come into their homes and who answered a questionnaire about their daily activities and use of services. Meeting the residents and finding out what they were doing was one of the most enjoyable parts of the research.

Lorna Wing and her research team, especially Dermott Bowler, have very kindly made some of their material available to us, and also spent time in discussion with us, sharing their perspectives on the project.

The research was funded by the Mental Handicap Research Liaison Group of the Department of Health and we are grateful to them for allowing us to follow through what was originally a three-year contract. During this time, they have maintained a keen interest in the project and have been supportive in a variety of ways. Special mention should be given to the two liaison officers who were involved with this project, Dr Sara Graham and Mrs Jenny Griffin, for their help, good advice and enthusiasm.

Our thanks as well to Geraldine Shaw, who cheerfully processed and reprocessed successive drafts of the manuscript at unsociable hours.

PART 1

The policy context

CHAPTER 1

Changing attitudes to institutions

During the second half of the nineteenth century, the Victorians turned their energies and reforming zeal to the facilities for those suffering from mental disorder. They built a series of large hospitals on the outskirts of centres of population. These large Victorian piles became a part of local landscapes and mythology. The quality of care found in them may have been poor by modern standards, but they did represent an improvement over the arbitrary and cruel treatment of individuals in private, unregistered madhouses which preceded them. Now, in the second half of the twentieth century, all this is being reversed. Institutions are seen as bad places, which harm rather than help their inmates. Deinstitutionalization is being taken up with the same fervour, rhetorical conviction and lack of experience that the institutional solution received in its time.

From the late 1950s, 'community care' became a bipartisan political objective, but 20 years went by before a major hospital closure was contemplated and nearly 40 years before it was achieved. The movement towards deinstitutionalization, transferring people from care in institutions to care in the community, began largely as ideology and has taken many years to translate into practice. This study seeks to explain why that has been so.

Creating institutions

It proved a great deal easier to build large institutions than it has been to dismantle them. The 1845 Lunatics Act made the establishment of asylums by county authorities compulsory. Jones and Scull provide opposing interpretations as to why asylums became a statutory obligation.

Kathleen Jones (1960) gives what might be termed a conventional interpretation of the history of mental institutions, emphasizing the humanitarian impulses behind the reform movement leading to the 1845 Lunatics Act. She cites the reports of the work of Metropolitan Commissioners between 1828 and 1845 which drew public attention to conditions in asylums. The County Asylums and Madhouse Acts had required regular visiting and inspection procedures and reports to the Home Department. The Lunatics Act extended the work of the Commissioners to cover the inspection of asylums and licensed madhouses throughout the country. The establishment of early institutions, such as the York Retreat and St Luke's in London, is described by Jones as arising from 'the consciousness felt by a small group of citizens of an overwhelming social evil in their midst' (p. 40). The evangelical and radical movements of the early nineteenth century and the growth of societies for the reform of particular abuses are shown to have contributed to the lunacy reform endeavours. Parliamentary select committees were active in drawing attention to poor conditions in workhouses and private madhouses. Scandals, too, contributed to the formation of public and political opinion leading to reform, in particular the fire at the York Asylum in 1813. Thus, in describing the Lunatics Act of 1845, Jones writes that 'Ashley and his colleagues had roused the conscience of mid-Victorian society, and had set a new standard of public morality by which the care of the helpless and degraded classes of the community was to be seen as a social responsibility' (p. 149). The model of government growth that is advanced by Jones is thus in the tradition of McDonagh's (1960) account of the passing of Passenger Acts in mid-Victorian England which regulated the transportation of migrants across the Atlantic in inhumane conditions. Public concern creates a public regulatory system whose inspectors expose more scandals and create pressure for more regulation and public provision.

An alternative explanation is provided by Andrew Scull (1979) in *Museums of Madness*. He argues that institutions were the outcome of urbanization, industrialization and professional forces that developed during the first half of the nineteenth century. (For a review of this study and a critical discussion of theories of social control and institutionalization, see Mayer, 1983, and Jones and Fowles, 1984.) The economic trends of the late eighteenth century – the development of a wage-based economy and low levels of wages resulting in a diminished capacity of the working classes to cope with loss of earnings – led to an increase in outdoor relief given by local parishes. The upper classes, however, believed that outdoor relief encouraged poverty by undermining low wages and sought a means of distinguishing the able-bodied from the non-able-bodied to force those who could do so to work. The indoor relief of the workhouse institution emerged as a solution to the need for such a practical test. It was an economic necessity to separate those who could not work from those who could and therefore should.

At the same time, ideas about lunacy were changing. It was becoming recognized as a loss of self-restraint and a sense of order, but not of humanity. This change of ideas was brought about in part by the exposures of the brutal treatment of the insane, and in turn made more humane treatment, re-education, resocialization and the abandonment of mechanical restraints, a more acceptable approach.

These changes in the values of society were paralleled by the rise of the medical profession. At the beginning of the nineteenth century, the medical profession were involved in the treatment of the mentally ill, but were far from exercising monopolistic control. Gradually, doctors successfully promoted themselves as the sole providers of treatment, claiming that mental illness was the outcome of disorders in the nervous system. Early detection and treatment of mental illness would lead to its being cured. The treatment proposed, however, was not a particularly medical one. It was the 'moral treatment' devised by Tuke which doctors argued would allow them to manage mentally ill people in large numbers, while avoiding the brutality and horrifying mechanical restraints which had been the source of public disquiet. With an optimistic faith in moral treatment, it was a comparatively easy step for the medical profession to encourage the public to transfer acceptance of workhouse institutions to separate institutions for lunatics.

A further argument in favour of separation was that of relieving the Poor Law institutions of undesirable and disruptive residents. This would allow the workhouse to be run properly, with no allowances needed for those who were obviously ill. The 1845 Act marked the triumph of the rising middle class – willing to support institutions for the ill but not unlimited outdoor relief for the work-shy, and concerned with order and discipline. Thus, Scull firmly places the reform movement in the context of the developing political economy of mid-Victorian society, and that is a valuable perspective. Yet it is only part of the story. Parker (1988) comments that 'Just as we need to justify why institutions gained or lost support as remedies for social ills we need to identify the reasons why, once established, some survived in the face of their objective failure to meet their aims.' Demography and economics are part of that story too.

The new institutions were almost immediately overwhelmed by the numbers of people with chronic illnesses referred to them and by local political pressure to keep costs down. Institutions were thus unable to fulfil the ideology of moral care and treatment which had made them initially acceptable to the public. Further, they came to be seen as catering for the pauper mentally ill who formed 90% of the asylum population. The increase in the number of mental asylums occurred at the same time as the number of workhouses was increasing, indicating the extent to which institutions were felt to provide relief to the community without necessarily giving relief to individuals (Skultans, 1978).

For people diagnosed as mentally deficient, the supposed link between mental deficiency and social problems – criminality, promiscuity – led to discussion of the need for sterilization and the segregation of people with mental deficiency. It strengthened the case for institutional care. These views were widely held in the last quarter of the nineteenth century and were based on what are now seen as suspect scientific claims advanced largely through the work of Sir Francis Galton, and authors of several studies of hereditary behaviour in families (Jones, 1960). Galton was noted for his work on eugenics, which purported to show that intelligence was as much an inherited quality as were physical characteristics. By implication, he argued that people of low intelligence would produce children of low intelligence, although his work actually produced no such evidence. This proposition seemed to be confirmed by Robert Dugdale in his study of the Jukes family in America, which traced the descendants of five mentally deficient sisters, showing a large proportion of them to be mentally deficient or antisocial (criminals, prostitutes, habitual paupers, etc.). A similar study was published in 1912 of the Kallikak family, showing similar results (Jones, 1960, p. 189). These ideas stirred up considerable public concern about how mental deficiency could be controlled. If it were inherited, then a policy of sterilization was appropriate for its prevention. On the other hand, it was unclear whether or not people with mental deficiency could be trained to live in the community, maintaining acceptable moral standards, in which case permanent segregation was not necessary.

The government set up a Royal Commission on the Care and Control of the Feeble-Minded (1904–1908) to examine these issues. One influential member was A. F. Tredgold, author of a major text on mental handicap (Tredgold, 1908) and member of the Eugenics Society which had campaigned for the segregation of 'defectives'. The Commission concluded that although heredity played some role in mental deficiency, and though mental deficiency was linked to some social problems, this was due to the freedom allowed to 'mental deficients' in the community. The Commission favoured a more stringent system of ascertainment and supervision which would protect the mentally deficient person. The Commission rejected a policy of sterilization. Its report laid the foundations for the 1913 Mental Deficiency Act, which recommended that each local authority establish a 'colony' as a basis for specialist custodial care. This would provide a completely self-contained and segregated environment where mentally deficient people of all ages could live, train, work and relax with villas for residences, schools, workshops, churches, recreational facilities and a farm. The First World War intervened to delay the construction of such 'colonies' until the 1920s and 1930s.

The issue of linkage between mental deficiency and social problems did not go away. The Wood Committee, established in 1929, was concerned primarily with the administration of mental deficiency services. It had come out strongly in favour of viewing services for mentally deficient people largely on the basis of social factors. It distinguished those capable of living a normal sociable life in the community under some form of supervision from those needing institutional care because of their antisocial or dangerous behaviour. The Committee made a distinction between primary and secondary amentia as causes of mental deficiency and thought only those whose mental deficiency was based on a primary cause, such as inherent genetic defects, represented the 'lowest tenth' of the population who needed to be segregated. Even those requiring care in segregated institutions needed care which would prepare them for life in the community (Jones, 1960, p. 224). The Committee again stressed the importance of the development of purpose-built colonies as the best means of caring for mentally subnormal people. Thus, many of the arguments used to justify the establishment of mental institutions in the mid-nineteenth century were used again to justify the establishment of separate institutions – the need for specialist facilities and for routines to control and classify people.

The period between the two wars saw the rapid expansion of specialized institutions for the mentally handicapped. Starting with 2040 such people in special institutions in 1914, the figure rose to 46 054 in 1939 (Alaszewski, 1986, pp. 14–15). By 1961, there were approximately 61 000 people in mental handicap hospitals. The number peaked during the mid-1960s to about 64 600 (Bone *et al.*, 1972).

The reaction against institutions

Just as the history of institutions is an interplay between the medical profession, public morality and hard political-economy, so too is the story of deinstitutionalization. Once again different authors emphasize different aspects of the story, but all the same elements are there in mirror image. Professional and public attitudes, scandal and the growing cost of maintaining these institutions began to produce a change in political perceptions. Finally, as the centenary of many of these institutions came and went the question of what to do with the outdated buildings and their increasingly valuable sites forced itself on to the hospital's and then health authorities' agendas.

Gradually, professional practice in the treatment of mental illness was beginning to change in ways which would eventually challenge the dominance and appropriateness of institutions as the desirable location of treatment for both mental illness and mental handicap. The open-door policy of mental hospitals – unlocking wards and keeping people as inpatients for only a limited period – began long before the introduction of psychotropic drugs in the mid-1950s, and was based on a recognition that keeping people in hospital for lengthy periods of time was detrimental to their ability to live once again in the community. Admission and discharge rates began to rise and total population of mental hospitals began to fall (Freeman and Farndale, 1963). This change, in turn, was related to other changes.

First, the growth of outpatient clinics and the inclusion of acute psychiatric wards as part of general hospitals began in the 1930s. It showed that treatment of mental illness was not synonymous with incarceration and helped to lessen its stigma. Changes in psychiatric practice during the Second World War – such as the development of group therapy, of methods of treatment without removal from everyday life, and of ideas that led to therapeutic communities – also helped to foster a more positive and active approach to treatment of mental illness. More generally, the spread of ideas associated with psychoanalysis began to blur the sharp division between normal and abnormal personality and behaviour and this too helped to destigmatize mental illness (Ramon, 1985).

The creation of the National Health Service (NHS) in 1948 and the involvement of post-war governments in a wider range of social problems brought issues of hospital care and mental disorders into the public domain. Many of these changes in practice occurred outside the large institutions, making them appear more rigid and hopeless in contrast.

A more direct assault on institutions, and on mental hospitals in particular, began in the early 1950s. One of the earliest issues concerned not conditions in institutions but the loss of liberty suffered by those wrongly certified and detained. *50,000 Outside the Law* (NCCL, 1951) rekindled fears about wrongful detention, which had in the previous century led to a legalistic process of certification for the mentally ill. This pamphlet argued that mentally subnormal people, as they were then called, lacked some of the legal safeguards available to the mentally ill against wrongful detention, and that the methods of testing young people for mental deficiency failed to distinguish temporary backwardness from permanent deficiency. Conditions in mental deficiency institutions created a 'vested interest' in retaining people rather than releasing them. Patients often did work which would otherwise require additional paid staff and hospitals took on commercial work without adequately paying patients. The pamphlet demanded a revision to existing law to prevent such conditions, and contributed towards the setting up of the Royal Commission on Mental Health in 1954.

Social scientists began to pay attention to state mental illness hospitals, starting with several studies carried out in America (Stanton and Schwarz, 1954; Belknap, 1956; Dunham and Weinberg, 1960). These studies and later ones tended to vary between aiming to modify circumstances within institutions and outright rejection of them. They focused on the interpersonal relationships among the various staff groups employed at the hospitals and between staff and patients. They examined how these special factors affected the prime objective of the hospitals, i.e. the care or rehabilitation of patients. What they claimed to have found was an organizational structure that encouraged custodial care rather than cure or rehabilitation. They found:

1 A considerable shortage of professional staff of all types within hospitals to carry out treatment programmes, which led to cynicism about their jobs and their role within the hospital.
2 Because of these shortages of staff, the treatment and management of patients was determined by the ward attendants, the least well-trained of all staff.
3 The extreme shortage of trained social workers resulted in poor links being maintained between patients and their families, and between the family, the community and the hospital, so that patients who might have been able to be discharged were left in hospital.
4 The social class differences between professional staff, especially doctors and attendants, led to attitudes of suspicion, avoidance and hostility, resulting in considerable barriers to communication. One author characterized the social structure of the hospital he studied as paranoid, with suspicion most apparent at the attendant level because of occupational and personal insecurities.

5 The differences between the formal and informal structures and objectives of hospitals were displayed most clearly at the ward level. The official duties of ward attendants, e.g. in the Southern State Hospital (Belknap, 1956), were to clean the ward and attend to the physical needs of the patients. However, the research revealed that due to understaffing (the hospital had 4800 patients and 600 staff), the ward attendants in fact spent their time supervising able patients who cleaned the ward, and washed and fed other patients – in short, most of the work that was officially the responsibility of the attendants. The large number of relatively able people in these hospitals were there to help on the wards – it was nothing to do with their welfare. The prime needs of the ward attendants were for order and control, and these tended to override the needs of patients.

In another study, Greenblatt *et al.* (1955) described how several hospitals had changed their regimes to produce therapeutic environments, underlining the importance of social rehabilitation as a key factor in the discharge process of mental illness hospitals. Mental hospitals came to be seen as preventing rather than providing treatment. These studies pointed to the importance of gaining the cooperation of patients in achieving their own recovery and of modifying the hospital environment so that it was more responsive to client needs than to organizational demands. Most of these studies attempted to find ways of making hospital care more effective. Only Belknap (1956, p. 205) challenged the ideology of hospitals outright: 'the failure of reform was to ask whether a large-scale, centralized and partly self-sufficient institution is in fact able to function effectively in the treatment of the mentally ill'.

The frontal assault on the underlying ideology of asylums was made by Goffman (1961). He analysed the social structure of institutions and the relations between inhabitants and staff, and introduced the influential concept of a 'total institution'. This was defined as 'a place of residence and work where a large number of like situated individuals, cut off from the wider society for an appreciable period of time, together lead an enclosed, formally administered round of life' (p. 11). The central feature of a total institution was said to be 'a breakdown of the barriers' found in ordinary life normally separating the place to live, the place to work and the place for recreation. Four characteristics of a total institution were cited:

- 'all aspects of life for the inmates carried on in the same place and under the same single authority';
- 'each phase of the member's daily activity is carried on in the immediate company of a large batch of others, all of whom are treated alike and are required to do the same thing together';
- 'all phases of the day's activity are tightly scheduled';
- 'the various enforced activities are brought together into a single rational purportedly designed to fulfill the official aims of the institution'. (p. 17)

Similar ideas were developed in England by, for example, Russell Barton (1959) in an extremely influential book *Institutional Neurosis*. Criticisms of mental hospitals in the UK were less strident and less condemning than those in America but, none the less, by the end of the 1950s and early 1960s 'progressive' thought in psychiatry was rapidly moving away from the hospital as a base for care towards the community. *Trends in the Mental Health Services* (Freeman and Farndale, 1963) brought together many of the leading exponents of community mental health and reproduced a number of influential articles, e.g. that by Tooth and Brooke which predicted that the number of psychiatric beds needed would fall from 3.4 per 1000 of the population in 1954 to about 1.8 for those admissions made in 1956. In their introduction, the editors noted that 'there is at present a period of tremendous upheaval, in which a system of care which has grown up over more than a century is being largely discarded' (ibid., p. x).

Similar trends in professional practice and dispute about institutional care spread through Europe. Reformers convinced politicians in some places but not others. The attack on institutions was not confined to mental hospitals. Other types of institution came to be seen as tarred by the same brush. Townsend (1962) carried out surveys of local authority, private and voluntary institutions for the elderly in England and Wales. His purpose was to describe the conditions found in institutions, and how elderly people lived in them. Townsend claimed that a significant proportion of the elderly then in institutional care had been admitted because of social factors rather than physical needs: homelessness, unavailability of domiciliary support services, financial insecurity, a general lack of social resources, of friends or family networks. Over half of new admissions, he claimed, were physically and mentally fit to lead independent lives.

What is so striking about his study are the descriptions of conditions in the homes – the management regimes, the social isolation of the inmates, their loss of occupation, the physical poverty of the environment, the loss of decision making by the elderly about their present life or future. Although not all institutions were rated as poor, the overall portrait presented was very grim.

A similar study of institutions for people with a mental handicap was produced seven years later by Pauline Morris (1969). She essentially extended the approach of Townsend to what were then called 'mental subnormality hospitals'. A comparably depressing picture emerged of meagre and inappropriate conditions. Two-thirds of the hospitals studied were housed in pre-1900 buildings. Only a minority of residents seemed to need hospital care – 65% of the patients had no physical handicap, 65% were able to dress and feed themselves, and only 12% were severely incontinent. The isolation of these hospitals affected staff as well as patients, and the shortage and lack of recognition of the value of specialist staff in education, occupational therapy and psychology, meant that only a small number of patients received any benefit from the supposed specialist service provided by hospitals. The stark contrast between the life led by patients in hospitals and the majority of adults in the community was due to loss of family contact, lack of activity for so many of the patients, crowded living conditions, and the treatment of residents by staff as if they were children. Even in voluntary homes, which were rated more highly than hospitals on standards of physical environment, the author claimed to have found few examples of rehabilitation or training.

A more strident attack on institutional care for the elderly was made in *Sans Everything* (Robb, 1967). The author based her claims on the evidence of several nurses working in geriatric units and the case of one elderly woman, the facts of which were subject to dispute. Callous indifference to patients, exploitation, rough handling, removal of glasses, hearing aids, dentures and other indignities, were portrayed as customary procedures. Although this pamphlet was scarcely of the same calibre as the research quoted above, it was rapidly followed by a series of revelations of cruelty and poor conditions in long-stay institutions in Britain which it may have helped to bring into the open. Because the pamphlet contained articles by a well-known consultant psychogeriatrician and an academic, it was given a degree of respectability which the evidence later showed to be unjustified.

Reports of inquiries set up to investigate allegations of ill-treatment became a feature of social policy literature during the 1970s. The best known is the report on Ely Hospital (DHSS, 1969). Others followed, continuing through to the report on Normansfield (DHSS, 1978). They presented a catalogue of failures at all levels of service provision and service management (Martin, 1984). In his analysis of reports by Committees of Inquiry into 19 hospitals, Martin cites the common features found in these hospitals which more or less mirror the sociological studies of hospitals in the 1950s: geographic and professional isolation; abandonment of patients by their communities; lack of support towards staff by management; failure of leadership among all professional groups and poor interaction and co-operation between professions; shortage of resources; 'corruption of care' – subversion of prime objectives of the hospital to the preservation of order, quiet and cleanliness. In the author's view, the failures of care were embedded in the social context in which the hospitals were run. Martin himself does not question whether so many or even any people should be in hospital. His recommendations are aimed at improving conditions within hospitals. But the series of hospital scandals which fomed the subject matter of his book publicized the negative features of hospital life the way no academic could, and largely contributed to the poor public image of hospitals.

Alternative services for people with a mental handicap were under-researched in comparison with mental illness. This perhaps reflected the belief dominant in the earlier part of this century that nothing could be done. The considerable change in attitudes towards mental illness seemed to pass by the services for mentally handicapped people. No move to run down these large hospitals appears in the Hospital Plan of 1962. Despite the general lack of academic interest, the MRC Social Psychiatry Research Unit was one research centre which examined the potential for development in people with a mental handicap. Several of their studies represent the first evidence of attempts to create alternative modes of provision. In passing, these studies were also critical of hospitals both for what they did and what they could do but did not.

O'Connor and Tizard (1956) reviewed studies relating to the ability of low dependency patients in hospital to work in ordinary employment situations. They described a series of experiments with hospital patients (some of which were carried out at Darenth Park) showing how rehabilitation services could be considerably improved. Their comments on training opportunities in hospitals highlighted how poor the rehabilitation services were (p. 91):

- most patients were given occupational activity rather than employed on work of value to the community;
- the work undertaken in hospitals had almost no relation to the kinds of jobs done on licence outside the hospital;
- equipment used in workshops was obsolete;
- little contact with commercial firms to take on trained people;
- the training situation was devoid of incentives;
- too little attention was paid to selection and training of supervisors and training staff;
- inadequate supervision of patients on licence or in daily service.

The authors argued that a far more effective service could be provided to enable many of the mentally handicapped to lead productive rather than dependent lives.

Further studies by Tizard (1964; Tizard and Grad, 1961) looked at the service needs of children with a mental handicap and their families and how services in the community could be organized to meet these needs. Tizard noted the ways in which attitudes towards residential care had changed after the Second World War and how the disadvantages of institutions had become increasingly apparent – their geographic remoteness; their intellectual remoteness from advances in medicine, education and psychology; the difficulties families faced in keeping in touch with their children. In particular, Tizard stressed the importance of size and its relation to the quality of service provided, picking up on a point made by Townsend in his study of residential care for the elderly.

A later study was concerned with the care offered to mentally handicapped children in institutions (King *et al.*, 1971). These researchers set out to examine how the environment of residential care provided influenced the way in which children were brought up, by comparing in detail the organization, staffing structures and patterns of daily activities in two local authority homes for children in care, one large paediatric hospital with long-stay wards and one mental subnormality hospital. Their conclusions supported many of the criticisms made of long-stay institutions. They claimed that they were not arguing against the size of institutions as such, but that size tended to be associated with other factors which worked against the interests of children, such as separation from the community, drawing residents from a wide area, making the retention of family and home links more difficult, greater problems in recruiting and retaining staff, and a greater tendency for centralization of organization within large institutions.

King *et al.*'s evidence (1971) showed how daily practices varied between and within the four institutions. The mental subnormality hospital adapted its care least to the degree of children's handicap. They pointed to the importance of the type of training the head of the unit received as critical to the mode of organization of the unit and noted that in terms of self-care and development of speech, mentally handicapped children in child-oriented units were more advanced than those in institution-oriented ones. Similar criticisms were made by Oswin (1974) in her study of weekend activities offered to handicapped children living in three different types of institution.

Another strand of psychological and sociological research examined families' coping strategies and the factors that precipitated entry to hospital. Tizard and Grad (1961) demonstrated that admission to hospitals for the mentally handicapped was less related to the needs of the person admitted but more to the family support system breaking down. Bayley (1973), in a sensitive study, described families' coping strategies, often adapting their lives in an extraordinary way to continue to care for a mentally handicapped child. They received very little help from statutory services – or very little the families found helpful. Family crisis and the ageing of the parents were the factors that resulted in hospital admissions. Hospital was the last resort: with more help hospitalization could be delayed and forms of care developed that were more like the family environment. This and other studies reinforced the view that family and family style care was a viable alternative to institutional care, if only the range of support was good enough.

More recently, a study by Booth (1985) examined the extent to which dependency of residents in local authority old people's homes is induced by the management regime of the home. He attempted to look at whether regimes induce dependency because of poor practice or whether an institutional setting is necessarily harmful, no matter what type of management style is adopted. Booth's study covered 175 homes in four local authorities over a two-year period. Despite finding differences in the 'ethos of regimes' (liberal to restrictive), the outcome for residents did not seem to vary according to regime. He concluded that 'sociologically, the differences between regimes must, in light of this study, be seen as a veneer that decorates the massive uniformity of institutional life . . . underneath lies the same crushing panoply of controls over lives and doings of residents' (p. 206). Even 'liberal' regimes did not avoid the negative effects of institutionalism: 'This study obliges us to face up to the fact that the only sure way of limiting its [residential care] harmful effects is to stop admitting people who, given the chance, could manage with other kinds of support' (p. 209). Similar conclusions are drawn by Willcocks *et al.* (1987).

Thus, to the political embarrassment caused by well-publicized scandals has been added a continuous stream of sociological research documenting the inherent difficulties of managing care in an institutional setting.

As a reaction to this negative analysis, sociologists and reformers produced their own alternative positive vision – 'normalization'. Tyne (1982) summarized the principles thus:

> . . . first, helping handicapped people to gain skills and characteristics, and to experience a life style which are valued in our society and to have opportunities for using skills and expressing individuality in choice; secondly, regardless of people's handicaps, providing services in settings and in ways which are valued in our society and supporting people to participate genuinely in the mainstream of life. This includes taking risks, carrying responsibilities and making choices; thirdly, by helping society to be much more accepting of peoples' differentness.

Much of the inspiration for this alternative principle of 'normal living' came from services developed in Nebraska in the USA. The Eastern Nebraska Community Office of Retardation (ENCOR) was the focus of many reformers' attention and its work was widely published in Britain by the Campaign for Mentally Handicapped People (1978) and the King's Fund (1980). Recent research on residential 'service' is reviewed by Atkinson (1988). We discuss the impact of this philosophy on policies in Chapter 2.

The political-economy argument

By itself none of this would have been enough to change the political climate. Almost 30 years of research and polemic had helped to create an intellectual climate in which institutions were seen as harmful to the interests and needs of their inhabitants. Yet little had happened to change the situation. Then, in the 1960s and 1970s, came the belief, strengthened by fiscal stress, that community care would be *cheaper* (Scull, 1984; Walker, 1982). Many of the hospitals, both in the UK and the USA, were 80–100 years old. If they continued to be used they would require major renovation or rebuilding. Closing them and selling their sites, on the other hand, would raise substantial capital revenues. Also, staffing these large unpopular hospitals in the 1960s had become a nightmare because of the short supply of labour. In the south-east of England, in particular, it could only be achieved by attracting labour from overseas to fill domestic and nursing positions in long-stay institutions. Those concerned with budgets saw that transferring people into the community would save revenue in several ways. Demands for improved standards in hospitals would require additional revenue, whereas decreasing the number of hospital patients would limit the numbers for whom services would need to be improved, and thus would limit the cost of improvement. Also, the National Health Service, faced with increasing financial pressures, saw that it would also be possible to shift the cost of care to local authorities, who were responsible for community care, or to families.

In the USA, similar financial incentives played a large part in developing programmes for discharging people from hospital. In the case of services in California, the interplay was between the state government (which supported the hospitals), local communities (which supported local services – health and welfare) and the federal government (which was willing to fund certain types of programmes but not others) (Segal and Aviram, 1978; Cameron, 1978). The same desire by the Federal Government to shift the fiscal burden is evident and is paralleled by a comparable policy in the case of the elderly (Estes *et al.*, 1983).

Doubts

Ideology, professional practice and economics combined to make deinstitutionalization a favoured option, just as they had a century before to create those very same institutions. But now, as then, the new policy has its critics. Brown *et al.* (1966) argued that the disabilities attributed to long stays in institutions were in fact, for some people, the symptoms of their illness. Discharge to the community would not change their characteristics and might make their condition worse by placing them in too demanding an environment. Jones *et al.* (1975) made a similar point with regard to people with a mental handicap. No theory of deinstitutionalization, normalization or labelling could deny the existence of severe handicaps and the need for special services. These critics challenged the assumption that institutions are always wrong for all people, and that the only types of disabilities are those acquired by living in an institution.

As in the nineteenth century, the demand for institutional care continued among those families who simply had no alternative (Anderson, 1971). Then, as now, the demand for institutional care was a fraction of the costs borne by families, the number of families affected and their capacity to cope on their own. Other critics based their doubts on more pragmatic considerations. Community care may be a viable alternative in principle they argued, but the facilities in the community were inadequate and thus deinstitutionalization as a policy was wrong because it encouraged discharge without adequate services. Sedgwick (1982, p. 192) argued that:

> in Britain as in the USA, the reduction in the register of patients resident in mental hospitals (from a peak of 154,000 in 1954 to around two-thirds of this total in recent years) has been achieved through the creation of a rhetoric of 'community care facilities', whose influence over policy on hospital admission and discharge has been particularly remarkable when one considers that they do not, in the actual world, exist.

None of this was new. Titmuss (1963) had from the beginning criticized the government for being too optimistic about the rundown of hospital beds. He argued that local authority expenditure on mental health services per head of population was less in 1959 than it was in 1951. He showed how various government policies conflicted with rehabilitation aims and warned that 'to scatter the mentally ill in the community before we have made provision for them is not a solution' (p. 223).

The most detailed documentation of the non-development of community services comes from the United States, and is more concerned with the mentally ill. Fears in Britain stem, in part, from that experience. In the USA, a new custodial private sector has grown up which provides alternative care for discharged patients – often unmonitored, and provided by unqualified staff. Some states have programmes that cater only for ex-hospital patients. Younger persons needing care, but having no record of hospitalization, are excluded. An increase in homelessness is linked with the growing number of ex-patients in what Brown (1985) calls 'the new marginality' – the way the public lumps together facilities for drug addicts, people with mental illness, convicts and other deviant groups. Brown, along with Chu and Trotter (1974), point to the way in which mental health programmes in the community are not necessarily linked with the mental health care needs of discharged residents. While it was in theory possible for new services to be created before old ones were dismantled, in reality this was rarely achieved in the USA (Bradley, 1976).

The Darenth Park Project was an explicit attempt to avoid these failures and provide adequate new local facilities. It was the first time such a large hospital would close in the UK. Would the British experience mirror that in the USA? We turn next to the national policy environment within which the local plans were developed.

CHAPTER 2

The national policy environment

We have seen that by the late 1960s a broad political and professional consensus had begun to emerge that 'something ought to be done about' the large long-stay hospitals for the mentally handicapped. Under the combined impact of the Ely Enquiry, Barbara Robb's campaigning skills and Pauline Morris' survey, people with a mental handicap were established for the first time on the national policy agenda. Richard Crossman, Secretary of State, set aside a capital allocation to encourage regional hospital boards, as they then were, to improve long-stay facilities. This was the forerunner of a more extensive policy to shift resources to the neglected client groups which became national policy in the mid-1970s (DHSS, 1976). Work began in the Department of Health and Social Security (DHSS) to prepare a national plan to develop services for the mentally handicapped not just within the National Health Service (NHS) but by local authorities too. A draft white paper was ready by the time of the general election in June 1970. The Labour Government lost office, but Sir Keith Joseph, the new Conservative Secretary of State, continued the initiative and published what was more or less the same document in March 1971, *Better Services for the Mentally Handicapped* (DHSS, 1971). This was the first detailed comprehensive guidance to be issued for any client group by a central department, and it became a model for subsequent white papers on the mentally ill (DHSS, 1975) and the elderly (DHSS, 1981d). As an approach to policy direction and implementation it fitted into the classic mould of what we have previously called 'the central rationalist model' (Glennerster *et al.*, 1983). The central department published a 20-year plan which set targets for health and local authority provision. There were recommended levels of provision per head of population in each sector. The core of the white paper was a programme for local authorities to develop residential and training places at the same time as a reduction in places provided within hospitals. In particular, it proposed:

- halving the hospital population over the 20-year period by an active discharge policy and the prevention of inappropriate admissions, notably of children;

- building smaller hospital units associated with general hospitals, units of 100–200 beds;
- improving existing hospital standards and staffing;
- expanding local authority provision of residential homes and day training places, which were to be nearly trebled;
- all able residents would be transferred to such care from existing hospitals, so that admissions would fall as these new facilities became available.

Like most government policy statements this built on existing experience. It disappointed the more radical proponents of community care. It did not refer to more far-reaching experiments that had taken place in Scandinavia or the USA. It was a compromise between those who would have liked to see almost all residents outside hospital care, and traditional medical and nursing interests who wished to retain significant hospital provision. The assumption was that the more able residents would become the responsibility of local authorities, and the more severely handicapped would remain in hospital, although in rather smaller and more modern ones. This was the view that informed the early planning stages of the Darenth Park Project.

Administrative and financial innovations

Central government created a number of innovatory mechanisms that were designed to push this plan forward. The first was devised in the wake of the Ely scandal. The purpose of the Hospital (later the Health) Advisory Service was to inspect and advise on standards of care in long-stay institutions, and it was to play an important role in the history of Darenth Park.

The second innovation was the National Development Group (NDG). In February 1975, a year after taking office, Mrs Barbara Castle, the new Secretary of State in the Labour Government, made what was in effect a major policy statement. She expressed disappointment with the slow response to community care outlined in the original white paper and announced the setting up of two new bodies, one of which was the National Development Group for the Mentally Handicapped. The role of this new body was to help fill out the policy detail within a broad set of principles. It was to last five years, and during that time published two bulletins, five pamphlets, a report on the mentally handicapped in hospital, a checklist of standards for improving the quality of services for mentally handicapped people, and a brief review of the Group's views on the way services should develop (NDG, 1980). The first pamphlet was entitled *Mental Handicap: Planning Together* (NDG, 1976), which presaged the advice contained in a circular on joint planning [HC(77)17] that the Department had issued four months earlier. The circular had suggested that when authorities set up joint care planning teams comprising health and local authority officers, membership should be extended to include people with specific knowledge of and interest in the service being planned. The theme of the second pamphlet, entitled *Mentally Handicapped Children: A Plan for Action* (NDG, 1977), was that community-based services for mentally handicapped children and their families should be improved. The concept of a community mental handicap team was developed in this pamphlet, though it had been mentioned in the first. The idea of these teams, composed of a core of two or three people with mental handicap nursing and social work experience, was not new but did receive considerable and important encouragement from the NDG. The NDG then went on to produce pamphlets on mentally handicapped school leavers, short-term care for mentally handicapped people, day services for the mentally handicapped and then, in October 1978, a report on helping mentally handicapped people in hospital. The last two publications of the group were both posthumous, appearing after the Group had been disbanded in April 1980. *Services for Mentally Handicapped People – Unfinished Business* (NDG, 1980) was more generally critical of policy and the allocation of resources for the mentally handicapped both by the Department and by local authorities. The NDG was disbanded in 1980 because, it has been suggested, central government had begun to find it embarrassing and it had lost the degree of ministerial protection that it had enjoyed until that date.

The third major innovation was the Development Team for the Mentally Handicapped which started work in 1976 and is still in existence, though now called the National Development Team for Mentally Handicapped People. It is a multidisciplinary group, backed up by a panel of people with experience in various aspects of mental handicap. It is available to advise individual health and local authorities and voluntary organizations over a whole range of planning, developmental and operational issues. The unique nature of this team has been that its brief has extended to commenting and advising on the range of services that were being provided jointly by the health and personal social services and voluntary organizations for the whole client group.

The fourth innovation has already been mentioned – a new form of funding called joint finance. The NHS could give money for a limited period to local authorities to encourage them to initiate new services which would in some way assist the NHS to achieve its objectives of community care. The mechanism was enshrined in two health circulars, HRC(74)19 and HC(77)17. It was small in extent and provided financial aid to local authorities which tapered off, leaving the local authority to pick up the long-term bill. Mental handicap services did proportionately well out of this new funding scheme, but it soon became apparent that although the principle was a good one, the fact that local authorities had to meet all the costs of the new services in the long term meant that it had only limited usefulness in funding major schemes of hospital closure. Despite the value of these innovations progress was disappointingly slow.

Constraints

The dramatic expansion in the early 1970s of local authority spending in general, and of the personal social services in particular, was to return to more sober levels after 1975. As the DHSS itself pointed out in a review of policy in 1980 (DHSS, 1980), the rate of growth in spending on health and personal social services fell from 4% in the early 1970s to 2% in 1974–5:

> The constraints since 1974, together with demographic pressures and the need to rationalise acute services . . . meant that health authorities could do little to sustain the previous increase in the expenditure of mental handicap services other than their increasing contribution through joint finance. [This] in its present form is not enough to bring about a major shift in the balance between health and social services for mentally handicapped people (DHSS, 1980, paras 6.16–6.20).

The DHSS's overall and diplomatic conclusion from this survey was that within existing public expenditure constraints 'the timetable for achieving white paper policies (let alone any further shift in care in the community) is likely to be a very long one'. In consequence, 'it would seem necessary to consider whether current strategy needed to be modified to bring it into line with public expenditure expectations and if so in what way?' As public expenditure constraints grew tighter after 1980, local health authorities were forced to use savings that they were making on acute services to meet efficiency savings demanded by the government, rather than being able to use the resources for priority groups. As the 1980s progressed, health authorities came under increasing pressure not to shift resources to the priority groups at all as more public attention and criticism focused on the deficiencies in the acute services. With the coming of the new Conservative administration in 1979 there was also a new attitude to central direction and planning. The assumptive worlds of policy makers in which the original white paper had been drafted no longer existed in the 1980s. It was not merely that notions of central planning came to be seen as outmoded, but the whole notion of collaboration as a feasible goal was also thrown into doubt by the hostility of many Labour local authorities to health authorities whom they saw being no more than a tool of the Conservative central government. The easy assumptions of collaboration and cooperation were no longer appropriate, if they ever were. Commenting on the overall progress of health and social service authorities towards the 1971 white paper objectives, the Audit Commission for Local Authorities (1987) described the greater pressures which were being exerted on local authorities to increase provision: the increasing number of adults with severe handicaps needing care, as a result of the successful medical treatment of severely handicapped children during the 1960s; the increase in life expectancy, in line with increased life expectancy of the general population; and the reduction of NHS short-stay and long-stay beds as part of reduction/closure programmes.

However, against this more gloomy scenario, other factors were at work.

A new start

A new philosophy of care

The Jay Report (DHSS, 1979), though primarily concerned with a new training strategy for staff, set out what at the time was a controversial statement of philosophy for the services. It incorporated many of the ideas of normalization mentioned in Chapter 1. The emphasis was on providing support for families with a handicapped member. Where alternatives to family or foster care were necessary the emphasis was on the provision of small, highly staffed units or on conventional housing. There was no place for the traditional long-stay hospital. Gradually, these goals came to influence local practitioners and managers. In its policy document *Care in the Community* (DHSS, 1981b), the new Conservative Government accepted the Jay Report with some reservations. In its later policy guidance the DHSS (1985) said:

> The Jay Report proposed a model of care under which those mentally handicapped people who need residential care away from home should receive this in small residential units, preferably in domestic housing, and sited in local communities, run either by health or local authorities. The Government accepted this in principle, but indicated the need for further consideration of the best way of providing for the special needs of the relatively small numbers of the most severely and multiply handicapped people. Thus health authorities should aim to accommodate eventually in small, homely units based in local communities all mentally handicapped people requiring care in a health setting, except possibly some special needs.

This statement essentially spelt the end for the long-stay hospital for mentally handicapped people.

A new set of financial incentives

In an attempt to resolve some of the financial and administrative difficulties that faced health authorities the DHSS produced a green paper setting out possible alternative ways to finance and administer the priority groups (DHSS, 1981b). These ranged from improving the rules for joint finance to setting up a new joint authority for each of the client groups. Eventually, new financial ground rules were created, some of which required additional legislation (the Health and Social Security Adjustments Act 1983). Two important circulars were published: HC(83)6 (DHSS, 1983b) and HC(84)9 (DHSS, 1984). It is worth spelling out the contents of these circulars because they were to affect the Darenth Park Project in important ways. Under their provisions:

1 District health authorities would be able to make continuing annual payments for as long as necessary to local authorities and voluntary organizations for people who were moving out of hospital into community care.
2 Joint finance could be paid for schemes to transfer people out of hospital for a period of up to 13 years with 100% support from the National Health Service for up to 10 years.
3 A programme of pilot projects was created and over £16 million allocated to develop and assess experimental projects.
4 Payments could be made by district health authorities for the support of education of handicapped people and for housing provided either by local authorities or by housing associations.

These new powers increased the freedom of health authorities to buy the collaboration of local agencies in assisting the process of hospital closure.

Normalization and new sources of funds

The philosophy of normal living not only provided a common basis for planning policy in many local areas, but it also had financial implications too. Residents who were to live in ordinary housing or hostels would, under social security regulations, receive social security payments, often at an enhanced rate. If these residents had remained in a state hospital, the full cost of their board and lodging would have fallen on the NHS. It was not surprising, therefore, that this new philosophy of care should appeal to local health service managers. Moreover, the new housing policy of the government also fitted fortuitously well into this new framework of care. The Conservative Government was even more anxious than its predecessor to encourage non-state housing associations. As part of their enormously complex system of grant support, housing associations were entitled to draw extra financial assistance if the association was providing hostel accommodation. Since philosophies of care increasingly favoured traditional housing, additional Exchequer funding through the Housing Corporation proved an attractive option. Thus while local authority budgets were being successfully squeezed, local health managers with an entrepreneurial spirit could arrange to relocate residents outside hospitals in such a way as to attract extra Exchequer assistance from non-NHS funds, both from the Housing Corporation and from the social security system. (See a letter from Len Peach and the NHS management board to Regional Chairmen dated 24 September 1987.) Understandably, government became worried by this trend, and it was one of the reasons for that second Griffiths Report on alternative ways of organizing and funding community care (DHSS, 1988).

Devolved managerial responsibility

From the time when the *Better Services* white paper was published by the

DHSS in 1971, the NHS was to pass through several phases of reorganization: the old regional hospital boards were replaced by health authorities in
1974; area health authorities were replaced by district health authorities in
1982; the districts restructured their units in 1982–3; and the new
management structures were replaced and a new breed of general managers
were introduced to run regions, districts and units in 1984. The individuals
responsible for carrying through service development strategies for the
mentally handicapped thus changed many times. This had some unfortunate
consequences. Nevertheless, on balance, changes which were introduced
after the first Griffiths Report on general management (DHSS, 1983a) did
prove an important contributory factor in speeding the process of hospital
closure in many areas. Unit general managers became key figures. Though a
great deal turned on the capacity of the particular individual involved, in
many instances it did create clearer lines of responsibility. It was, moreover,
in a manager's career interest to see that something happened. One person
could be held responsible for developing services for the mentally handicapped in an area faced with hospital closure. Thus, after a period of
uncertainty and disruption caused by the coming of general management, the
outcome in many districts was beneficial to the programme of reprovision. So
it was to the process of hospital closure. A single person could be given charge
of the complex process of running down a large institution.

Pressure from above

As part of the same process of reorganization, central government introduced
a procedure of accountability reviews. Under this system, regions and
districts had to respond to questions from the central department about their
progress towards key policy goals. Mental handicap and the closure of
long-stay institutions featured as one of those key policy areas on which
managers had to report progress.

In parallel with this, the Audit Commission brought pressure to bear on
local authorities. It followed up a critical report on the organization of
community care (Audit Commission, 1986) with an occasional paper which
was entirely devoted to giving advice to local authorities about expanding
provision for the mentally handicapped (Audit Commission, 1987). This
paper was to provide the basis for auditors from the Audit Commission to ask
questions of local authorities about their policy for the mentally handicapped. The paper pointed out that, as the NHS reduced its provision of
long-stay places in hospital, the burden on local authorities would increase. It
went on:

> This process of change appears set to accelerate. Many health authorities
> now have plans to close long stay hospitals within the next ten years, and
> at least two regions are hoping to close all of their provision in that time
> period. If these targets are to be realised, there will need to be a
> considerable increase in the rate of resettlement, and the people actually

being resettled will inevitably be older and more dependent. Health authorities face major problems as a result and bridging finance is needed if satisfactory alternatives are to be developed.

The implications of these developments need to be addressed urgently and require a coordinated approach with health authorities (paras 17 and 18).

During 1988 the Commission's Auditors intend to undertake local audits of personal social services for people with a mental handicap and will be looking to see how authorities are meeting these requirements (para. 65).

In short, pressure was being brought to bear by central government on both district health authorities and on their local authority counterparts.

Doubts remain

Despite the fact that hospital closure was now a high priority for health authorities, public doubts remained. In January 1985, after a hearing that lasted seven months, the House of Commons Social Services Committee published what was to be a very influential report (House of Commons, 1985). It represented the first official evidence of some backlash against hospital closure, not least a more wary attitude to the pace of hospital closure, and fears about the level of alternative provision that was being made. The Committee's concerns were encapsulated in a key passage:

Earlier community care policies were embarked upon in the apparent belief that it was the institutions that created many of the disabilities of those within them and that modern medical and psychological techniques would lead to a massive reduction in the need for long term care. There are now only vestiges of such a blithely over-optimistic attitude . . . there is a growing recognition that 'institutions' – meaning primarily hospitals – may have fulfilled at least one function that has to be replicated if they are to be replaced: that of 'asylum', by which is meant the provision of shelter and refuge (para. 25).

That did not mean, the Committee argued, relying on 'vast institutions':

Asylum can be provided in a physical and psychological sense in the middle of a normal residential community . . . but we must face the fact that some people need asylum (para. 26).

For all these reasons, as the Committee itself pointed out, proper evaluation of hospital closure is important. The Darenth Park Steering Group, which played an overseeing role in the closure process, had the foresight to provide for a continuous evaluation of the process of closure and the DHSS supported the research. In Chapter 3 we describe the origins of the closure, plans and an overview of the period during which the closure was carried through. This will enable the reader to follow the more detailed discussion of the policy process at local level which follows later.

PART 2

The administrative politics
of closure

The Darenth Park project: early history and overview

Darenth Park Hospital

Darenth Park was one of the oldest institutions in England built specifically for people with a mental handicap. The changes of name it underwent during its existence reflected the changing public attitudes to the care and treatment of mental handicap. It began as 'Darenth School' for 500 children in 1878. However, it soon found itself unable to place the children back in the community, and 10 years after it was founded, it accommodated over 1000 adults *and* children. In 1911, Darenth School became the 'Darenth Industrial Training Colony', offering domestic, agricultural and industrial training for men and women. The colony was just about self-sufficient, providing much of its own food, furniture and clothing. It had its own water and gas supplies. In 1919, its name was changed to the 'Darenth Training Colony', with an emphasis on the training of 'high-grade defectives'. In 1936, the name was changed again to 'Darenth Park Hospital', at the same time as it was transferred to the London County Council (LCC). In 1948 its management was taken over by the NHS.

In 1934, Darenth stopped admitting children, because other services for children in the area had begun to develop and the numbers at Darenth were declining. However, short-term care admissions for children began again in 1952, and long-term admissions in 1954. The former change was in response to a central government circular, and the latter to local demands. In the early 1960s, the Regional Hospital Board (RHB) made special provisions for children with mental handicap at Goldie Leigh Hospital in Greenwich, originally built as an orphanage in 1902 by the Woolwich Board of Guardians. It had then become, during the First World War, a hospital for children suffering from skin diseases. The use of Goldie Leigh for children from the catchment area meant that the only children at Darenth Park were from the Dartford area. When children at Goldie Leigh reached the age of 16 or so, the policy was for them to transfer to the adult facilities at Darenth Park.

Located on the outskirts of Dartford, Kent, the hospital had traditionally taken people primarily from the London area but had also occasionally

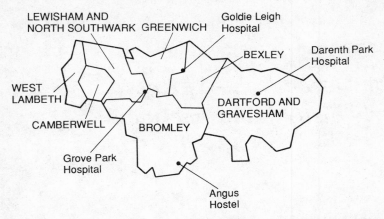

Figure 3.1 The catchment area for Darenth Park Hospital and residential facilities for mentally handicapped adults, 1978.

accepted people from the rest of England. In the early 1960s, the hospital was given a defined catchment area for the first time: the five London boroughs of Lambeth, Southwark, Lewisham, Greenwich and Bexley and the north-west part of Kent in which the hospital was located. Eight or so years later, the RHB included Bromley in Darenth Park's catchment area to try to relieve severe overcrowding at the second large mental handicap hospital in the region, Leybourne Grange (see Fig. 3.1 for a map of the area and the administrative boundaries).

The defined catchment area of the hospital contained quite diverse features. Politically, the area ranged from strong left-wing Labour councils in the inner-London districts to suburban Tories in Bexley and Bromley and shire Tories in Kent. The political complexities of councils had a significant impact on the Darenth Park Project – it coloured attitudes towards relations with health authorities, towards working with private and voluntary organizations including housing associations, and towards a general willingness to develop services. The various struggles with central government over constraints on local government finance diverted the attention of Labour authorities from service developments, but the constraints on finance would have limited that in any case, with districts adopting different management styles and models of service provision.

Another important difference within the catchment area was the balance between private and public sector housing and the influence this had on the capacity of districts to find properties suitable for group homes (see Table 3.1). The greater share of public sector housing in inner London should have made it more difficult finding properties, but this factor does not appear to have been a major problem and was balanced by the much higher cost of properties in the suburbs.

The inner-London districts had a wider variety of active voluntary organizations to involve in both planning and service provision than existed

Table 3.1 The housing stock in the catchment boroughs[a]

	In public sector (including housing associations) (%)	In private sector (%)
Bromley	17	83
Bexley	20	80
Greenwich	47	53
Lewisham	49	51
Lambeth	54	46
Southwark	74	26

[a] Taken from Table 117, Housing Stock by Section in Greater London April 1986. *Annual Abstracts of Greater London Statistics*, 1986/87. Vol. 19, London Research Centre, London.

in the suburbs, including more local branches of national voluntary organizations, parents' groups, a university settlement and other groups. This partially reflected the active encouragement given to such organizations by their local authorities – financial support, working party involvement and access to council committee meetings and officer time for advice and development.

The social and physical environment thus varied considerably: it showed in the style of clothing people wore (Levis *vs* suits for social services staff) and in the street culture – two very different worlds.

Among the first of the public purpose-built institutions for people with a mental handicap, Darenth Park has also been among the first of such institutions to close, and was certainly the first large hospital to close. It was achieved without transferring those residents with 'challenging behaviour' to another hospital. New and innovative services have been developed which aim to allow everyone to live in the community.

The first serious discussion of closure dates back to the early 1970s. Actual closure was achieved in August 1988. Parents and staff were less enthusiastic about a change of service. There followed years of trying both to improve conditions at Darenth Park, which achieved very little, and to develop new facilities in the districts using the hospital. In the end, although the Darenth Park Steering Group, which saw through the project, sat for 10 years, most of the innovation in administrative techniques and service development actually took place during the last five years of the project, from 1983 to 1988. We shall explore why this was so.

The 1970s

In the year that the report on conditions in Ely Hospital was published, Darenth Park Hospital had approximately 1500 residents. The hospital had more than 40 wards, of which 10 contained more than 50 residents. Ten wards were single-storey pavilion wards; the rest were in two- and three-storey ward blocks, one male corridor, one female corridor. Long after the wards became mixed sex, the corridor names remained in use.

In response to the Ely Report, regional officers visited the hospital and began drawing up plans for improvements to living and working conditions there. Before much could be done, the Hospital Advisory Service (HAS) visited in February 1970, and again in October of that year. Poor communication between staff at different organizational levels and between different staff groups at all levels was a prime finding of their visits. A specific recommendation was that the wards, then organized in relation to the abilities of residents, be reorganized on the basis of local authorities, so that each consultant and his medical and nursing team would deal with residents with an entire range of abilities from one designated locality.

This 'sectorization' of the hospital into groups of wards matching the local authorities from which residents came took seven years to achieve. The consultant staff were most resistant to change. The hospital had to acquire a fifth consultant to give more or less even distribution between wards. The aim behind sectorization was to make it easier for local authorities to work with their own residents in the hospital, all of whom would now be grouped together, and it was hoped this would lead to easier discharge. However, this did not happen.

Social work support was the responsibility of the local authority in which the hospital was located. What few social workers there were assigned to the hospital came from Kent County Council. They would not take most of the residents. The other local authorities refused to be involved. Thus sectorization did not bring local authorities into the hospital. Indeed, it created two additional problems for the health service which later affected the Darenth Park Project. First, District Health Authority (DHA) boundaries were not the same as the local authority boundaries. Yet it was the DHAs who would have the responsibility for moving residents out. A simple course in Social Administration here might have helped! Secondly, sectorization disturbed many friendships as residents were redistributed among the sectors on the basis of area of origin. When residents were allocated to districts at a later stage, district officers sought to get friends back together again.

A second recommendation of the HAS report was that the Regional Hospital Board give serious consideration to closing Darenth Park. Its buildings were simply not able to allow more modern methods of care to be given. Regional officers took this point seriously. Although they could not agree to hospital closure immediately (a radical thought in 1970), they accepted that it would, at least, be an improvement to transfer some of the residents off site. They therefore began to look for places in the London area which could accommodate a significant number of residents, and settled for Grove Park Hospital.

Grove Park had been built in the 1890s as a tuberculosis hospital. It was located in about 15 acres of land, through which ran the boundary between

Lewisham and Bromley. It was then being used as a chest, geriatric and thoracic surgery hospital, but it had unused beds. It seemed a simple proposition to transfer those patients to other hospitals and have the entire space available for Darenth Park residents. Grove Park presented certain advantages. First, it was NHS property available for NHS use. Secondly, sites in London were always hard to find, certainly of that size. Thirdly, it would recruit nursing and domestic staff far enough away from Darenth Park so as not to compete with it. Fourthly, the reduced distance to London meant that it was significantly easier for relatives to keep in touch with family members in the hospital. Finally, because of the size of the site, it could not only accommodate residents in existing buildings, but it would permit the construction of purpose-built units for residents of Lewisham and Bromley.

Thus at the end of 1970, regional officers embarked upon what was intended to be a quick upgrading (largely redecoration) of existing wards at Grove Park. In reality it turned into a 10-year project. Local health service officers and works officers demanded high standards of conversion. Difficulties ensued, entirely predictable when an old building is tampered with, e.g. new fire regulations came into effect which necessitated additional work, and asbestos was found in service ducts which needed to be removed. The final wards of this 'temporary solution' did not open until 1981. The new permanent units never got planning permission from Bromley Council, the excuse being that the hospital was in 'green-chain' land where new development was restricted.

Throughout the 1970s, regional officers maintained their interest in improving conditions at Darenth Park. Various studies were undertaken to show how many residents would remain by the end of the decade and what facilities they would need. Kent County Council was approached to take over some of Darenth Park's wards and to run them as hostel facilities, to cater for the large number of residents with very mild mental handicap. As a result of a review of conditions in Darenth Park in 1972 by a team of regional officers, plans were drawn up to upgrade the least satisfactory of the wards, increasing nursing and domestic staff, providing new specialized facilities, and recruiting more remedial therapy staff. Their report led directly to the RHB's agreement in January 1973 to work for the closure of Darenth Park, although over a very long period of time, because capital was not available for total replacement.

Another working party was set up in 1976 to review what had happened so far at Darenth Park, and to decide what the next steps were to be. A liaison group was established, also in 1976, with the social services departments using the hospital as a means of improving communication and encouraging more discharges. Neither of these objectives were achieved.

One of the reasons closure kept slipping from the Region's agenda was its shortage of capital. Plans were made but rarely implemented because they were too optimistic in relation to the likely capital building programme. Yet the costs of renovation at Grove Park kept eating up what capital was available for mental handicap provision.

The approach from Blue Circle

Towards the middle of the 1970s, regional officers were approached by the Blue Circle Cement Company with a view to the company buying Darenth Park Hospital because of the chalk which lay underneath the main hospital buildings. The chalk was worth only £2–3 million, but Blue Circle was willing to pay much more because of the proximity of the chalk to a newly built processing plant in the area. The chalk was needed to keep the plant fully operational. The Region saw the attraction of selling the hospital: here was the means of acquiring enough capital to actually provide for the complete replacement of Darenth Park. However, people living in the area did not see this in the same light: there were already several excavation sites in the area, and thus the issue went to a public planning enquiry in April 1978.

The Darenth Park Steering Group

If the public enquiry decided in favour of Blue Circle, the hospital site would have to be vacated by 1 January 1985, just six and a half years ahead. In order to be able to comply with this condition, the Region decided to plan for that timetable and in June 1978 convened the first meeting of the 'Darenth Park Steering Group'.

Membership of the Steering Group, in additional to regional officers, consisted of representatives of the four area health authorities involved, the hospital, the health district in which the hospital was located, and two Directors of Social Services, representing the seven directors of local authority social services in the catchment area. Initially, the Steering Group met monthly, as it needed to proceed with haste. In its evidence to the public enquiry two months earlier, the Region had indicated its plans for alternative accommodation. These consisted of providing one unit per district with a day centre and staff accommodation on site. DHSS (1971) norms indicated that no district would require more than 180 places, well within the *Better Services* guidelines of no more than 200 residents on one site. Further, regional officers, architects and works departments had been involved for several years in producing a standard design for mental handicap units which would incorporate some of the ideas found in *Better Services* (especially more domestic environments) and be within the cost limits. This design could now be advanced and made available to all districts, whose needs for new facilities would be similar. This way of proceeding would economize on planning time, effort and staff, major concerns to the Region. Standard units from the drawing board could be sited in each district. That was the hope.

The early meetings of the Steering Group and discussions with area officers outside these meetings showed that this service model was unlikely to win approval. Earlier the Region might have been able to impose its views on service development on areas and districts; however, the new NHS planning system (DHSS, 1976) required consultation in the planning process. In-formally, it was made known to the Region that districts did not like what regional officers were proposing. District officers saw the plan as simply shifting the institution from Dartford to new local sites. It represented a centralized style of service. In short, areas and districts were unlikely to accept it. Pragmatically, it was also dubious whether sites of sufficient size could be found in each district.

The Capital Planning Group, a sub-group of the Darenth Park Steering Group consisting of regional officers involved in planning, came up with a compromise model. Regional officers wanted to retain the economies of scale in planning which a uniform model for each district would achieve, yet accepted that they needed to meet some of the local objections in order to get agreement to proceed. The Capital Planning Group recognized that a consensus did not yet exist as to the best way of providing services for people with a mental handicap. It accepted that it needed to provide a model which was more flexible than the first, one which could adapt to changing needs. The new model consisted of a residential centre for each district, catering for about 72 residents in houses or flats with a day centre on site. The remaining places needed in districts would be provided in 24-place hostels in separate locations.

Some of the districts accepted the Steering Group's guidance – Bromley, Dartford and Gravesham (planning had already begun in 1977 for a replacement unit for the district's mental handicap services), King's (now Camberwell), Greenwich and Bexley, although in the latter two cases, difficulties were experienced over adequate sites. Lewisham, already having Grove Park Hospital, did not need to plan any further facilities.

At the end of 1979, the public enquiry resulted in permission for the extraction of chalk being refused. Although intensely disappointing, the Darenth Park Steering Group – local authorities included – agreed to carry on planning for the closure of Darenth Park as so much momentum had already been built up. It was, of course, recognized that the closure would take place over a longer time-span because of the loss of external capital.

By 1982, when NHS restructuring removed the area tier, some progress had been made over the plans in Bromley, Dartford and Gravesham, Greenwich, and Camberwell. The planning model had been accepted in Bexley but no site was available. St Thomas's (now West Lambeth) and Guys (now part of Lewisham and North Southwark) both rejected the planning guidance. Guys had set up its own development group for mental handicap services and was intending to provide services on a core and cluster model. St Thomas's intended to develop community services first, so that there would be a network of services for residents to come back to. But by 1982, only about half of the Darenth Park residents had been placed in alternative community accommodation – and these were still in the planning stage. Without further progress, the hospital could not close.

Local authority involvement

Progress with local authorities fared little better. It was originally hoped that the Darenth Park Project would be a joint planning exercise, resulting in those Darenth Park residents not requiring health services care being transferred to the care of local authorities. However, this did not work out, largely, but not solely, because of finance. The local authorities suspected the Region would profit from the Darenth Park site, and wanted to be certain that in taking over some responsibility they would receive adequate funding. When the sale of the site fell through, the local authorities still requested that the Region provide the full capital and revenue costs of service provision, without which they would not be willing to participate. Further, they wanted this to be 'new' money, that is, something besides the joint finance they saw as being intended for people already living in the community.

In 1981, one of the local authorities put up a test case. It offered to purchase a house and use it for residents from Darenth Park, provided all costs were met. When the Region refused to alter its views, local authority representatives walked out and withdrew from the Steering Group.

A second, far less dramatic but equally important explanation for the absence of joint planning was the actual approach used by the Region. In issuing guidance for the planning of the replacement facilities, the Region initially requested areas to produce plans for mental handicap services agreed with their local authorities within two months. This exercise in fact took almost a year. These plans related only to NHS provision for replacement services, and therefore left large areas of service provision to be negotiated separately. But this method of planning actually injected a fair degree of tension into the relationship: no authority likes to be pressured into an immediate decision. On the other hand, regional officers were aware of the shortage of time before the hospital site had to be vacated. Later, the planning guidance which put forward a model of care in effect cut across local efforts at joint planning by removing several of the key issues from local planning, e.g. the number of places the NHS should provide, and the types of facilities to be provided. Two local authorities seemed to adopt the view that as long as the NHS did not make demands on them for services, whatever they planned would be acceptable to them. In the others, the need for speed, coupled with NHS determination to go ahead anyway, soured a collaborative relationship.

A fresh start

By the time the NHS was restructured in 1982, regional officers were becoming increasingly concerned about the Darenth Park Project. Plans for only about 400 places had progressed enough to get into the capital programme. This represented about 60% of the number of places the region thought it would need to provide for the hospital to close. Restructuring had brought into the districts staff who were less content to follow the Steering Group guidelines on service development, and more responsive to the emerging ideology of normalization.

Until 1982, the Region had been in direct contact with area authority officers. However, they were now abolished in the NHS reorganization and contact had to be re-established with a new set of district officers who would now be directly responsible. Area staff had always been at one stage removed from service provision.

The Region still had to achieve several basic objectives: getting commitment from each district to the closure of Darenth Park; getting agreement among districts as to how many residents each district would accept and, as part of that, how many non-catchment residents each district would accept; and finding ways for the Region to provide funds to districts to pay for new services when the region's own development funds were being cut.

District agreement

Requests from the hospital for money to upgrade the building provided a clinching argument that persuaded districts. The sums involved were so large that the Region would have to slice off a part of all districts' funds to pay for it. The same money distributed among the catchment districts would enable them to fund local provisions. Nobody was prepared to argue that it was wise to spend so much on the hospital and a tentative closure date of 1 April 1987 was reached.

A new funding policy

In May 1983, the region produced a new funding policy for mental handicap services. This was based on a 'dowry' system. Districts would receive an annual sum of revenue per discharged resident, regardless of degree of handicap. It applied to all multidistrict mental handicap hospitals in the region and to all districts – not only those in the Darenth Park catchment area – who were taking residents out of hospital. It represented 'new' money to districts. It was not taken from joint finance and was additional to existing district revenue. The policy was linked to the government's *Care in the Community* (DHSS, 1981b) circular, which permitted the transfer of revenue to local authorities and voluntary organizations providing the care (for more details see Chapter 4).

Specialist staff to prepare for closure

The capacity of the Region to resolve other problems was assisted by changes which took place at the regional level itself. At the end of 1983, a regional staff training co-ordinator was appointed, a joint appointment between the RHA and Kent University. The person appointed had previously been involved in working and living in ordinary housing with people with severe mental handicap. Now, for the first time, the Region had someone on its staff who had experience of the new type of service, one which was only just beginning to spread. With that experience, the training co-ordinator was able to build confidence that it was possible to provide locally based services to cope with the most severe forms of handicap. His confidence was used by other regional officers to support changes in the direction in which development in Darenth Park were about to take. Regional officers now had professional care justifications for change.

The Region also gained a mental handicap planning co-ordinator in April 1984. Previously, no extra administrative support was available to the Darenth Park Project. This was one of the reasons why progress had ground to a halt. One of the first tasks undertaken by the mental handicap planning co-ordinator was to review the capital programme and see what could be done to speed things up.

A new form of provision

Experience showed that purpose-built facilities being planned and constructed by the Region were taking many years to complete. The Steering Group had already agreed to aim to close Darenth Park by 1 April 1987. If the facilities needed to reaccommodate the remaining residents in Darenth Park followed the existing pattern, there was no way this deadline could be met, and therefore the mental handicap planning co-ordinator had to convince the Region that a housing programme based on working with housing associations and using housing stock in the community was not only possible but was the Region's only chance of moving quickly enough to have new services ready on time. A housing programme emerged within 18 months.

Allocating residents

It was still necessary to decide how many residents, including non-catchment residents, each district would take. Some districts were having difficulty finding adequate sites or houses for the number of residents for whom they were responsible. Other districts were willing to take a greater number of residents than they were being asked to accommodate, provided they were given the necessary additional funding. The new funding policy made it possible to be more flexible in negotiating new agreements on the number of residents for districts.

Special Needs Policy

Some residents posed particular difficulties for districts. It had been made clear to districts that they would be expected to care for clients with severe mental handicap and severe behaviour problems in district facilities but a small working group was set up by the Regional Steering Group to look at ways of caring for similar clients in Leybourne Grange Hospital. This Group eventually agreed that a small unit was not really viable and proposed the establishment of a Regional Special Development Team to work with staff in local settings, caring for these clients. The team was to have five or six members from a variety of disciplines – nursing, social work, psychology, education, etc. The team was to assess clients referred to them by districts and produce a plan of recommended services, including accommodation required by the client. The districts were to implement these recommendations, using some additional funds made available by the Region. The team became linked to Kent University, in part to allow all of its staff to be employed on the same salary scales, something which would have been impossible if they were employed by the NHS.

For those clients with a mild mental handicap and challenging behaviour a unit was to be established which could assess psychiatric and psychological aspects of individuals' behaviour and advise districts on what would constitute good programmes of care for them. The new Special Needs Policy was approved by the RHA in April 1985.

The proposal for an assessment and treatment unit for people with a mild mental handicap and severe behaviour problems presented some difficulty to regional officers. They preferred to see services localized rather than centralized in a special unit. Also, they had no arrangements for a special unit or an alternative to it, but were quite determined that a service had to be developed because they would not allow Darenth Park residents to transfer to other hospitals. The special health authority centred on the Maudsley took up the idea of an active treatment unit. It had the facilities and expertise – all it lacked was money. In line with the regional viewpoint was the fact that the Maudsley was unwilling to provide long-term care. It was only interested in a treatment and discharge service. Months of negotiation, largely over costs, eventually resulted in the establishment of the Mental Impairment Evaluation and Treatment Service (MIETS) in a separate ward block at the Bethlem Royal Hospital, which took its first residents in May 1987.

The third strand to the special needs policy concerned people with sensory handicaps. This was the least developed of the special needs policies, and there was an amount of uncertainty as to the needs for services and the ways in which they could be met. As a first step, a development worker was appointed in early 1988, funded equally by Region, the DHSS and the Committee for the Multiply Handicapped/Blind, an umbrella organization for several organizations linked loosely to the Royal National Institute for the Blind. The task of the development worker was to gather information and make proposals about how the needs of the visually impaired could be approached. Secondly, the development worker was to promote local initiatives. The first of these, funded by the Region, was sponsored by Lewisham and North Southwark. It provided an audiology service for people with a mental handicap. The health authority had already established, through a pilot study of 100 people, that there was a very high incidence (80%) of untreated or incorrectly treated hearing loss in people with a mental handicap. The new project aimed to improve the take up of hearing aids and treatments for hearing disorders among people with a mental handicap, link this in with a speech therapy service and evaluate the effects of treatment on speech development and other areas of life. The project began in 1988 and is to last three years.

For the Darenth Park Project the timing of the establishment of the Special Development Team proved difficult. The team members, who were appointed during the first half of 1986, were to take referrals from the districts, make assessments and decide which of the referrals they would accept. Next, the team had to devise programmes (an individual service plan) for clients and present them to the district for approval. In general, the team recommended that clients referred to them live with one or two others who did not present challenging behaviours. These recommendations needed to be accepted by districts. However, by this stage, most districts had already decided on how to group their clients, and so the proposals caused some disruption to existing plans. The relatives of clients needed to be consulted, and their agreement sought; however, this was not always forthcoming. Very often, the recommendations for residential arrangements required district funding, finding additional houses and recruiting staff specifically for this type of project. Finally, there were negotiations about the costs of such a service. Even with the regional subsidy for these services, contributions required from the district were often above the level of the dowry. For these districts in the Darenth Park area, the Special Development Team came late in the day, and several of the team's clients were among the last to leave Darenth Park.

Consultation on closure

Formally speaking, in February 1985 the Darenth Park Steering Group discussed the results of its consultation on the closure. A document produced by Dartford and Gravesham Health Authority had been sent to all local authorities and district health authorities using the hospital asking for their views. This perhaps was made easier by an NDT report issued in January 1984 which urged all mental handicap hospitals in Kent to be closed because they were too old and too unsuitable for modern care. Objections to the closure document largely concerned the need for assurances about the maintenance of adequate care standards in the hospital before closure and in the new facilities in the districts after closure. However, soundings taken at this stage of the project made nonsense of the consultation process. The hospital was closing and agreement was the only realistic response.

The final stages

By the end of 1984 there were still about 160 places yet to be found for Darenth Park residents. The Region set up a task force, whose work was to ensure that the search for and acquisition of properties was speeded up. The task force membership brought together key regional personnel concerned with progressing the various aspects of the Darenth Park Project – planning, finance, architect's department and works. It was chaired by the regional nursing officer, who was also Chairman of the Darenth Park Steering Group. The task force, by bringing together the key people on a regular basis, helped to overcome many of the obstacles which occurred in the final three years, and provided support to regional officers who often came under considerable pressure. It was both a working group and provided moral support.

The result of the task force and the increased emphasis on housing led to the Region seeking a more collaborative agreement with the Housing Corporation and housing associations. A seminar on housing was held in September 1985 to inform districts about the complex procedures involved. It led eventually to a streamlining of approval procedures by the various regional departments. From 1985 onwards, each Steering Group meeting received a listing of all the proposed properties in each district and their target dates for completion. This paper formed the basis for the monitoring by the Region and could be used by the hospital to estimate what run down in its facilities would be needed. Two major issues remained – to provide for those with challenging behaviours and to resolve what to do with those residents who had not yet been allocated to districts.

The special needs policy for the first group has already been described. This left those residents who had not been allocated to a district. In most cases they presented no problem. A district simply took those residents who had no formal link with the district but were already residing in the wards of their sector. When districts shared wards on a sector (for example, North Southwark, Camberwell and West Lambeth shared the wards of the Lambeth/Southwark sector) the process took longer. Bromley Health Authority agreed to take non-catchment residents from the Greenwich/ Bexley wards to meet its target number of residents. However, by 1985 there were still about 50 residents who had not been allocated to a district.

The names of the non-allocated residents were divided into two groups. One group consisted of those who had challenging behaviours and would require special arrangements, or simply higher staffing levels. No district volunteered to take these residents. At the end of 1986, the regional nursing officer asked the consultant psychiatrist associated with the Mental Impairment Evaluation Team at the Bethlem Hospital and the leader of the Special Development Team to assess each resident from case notes and produce a profile of those 16 residents with special needs. In January 1987, the Darenth Park Steering Group meeting was devoted to ensuring that those residents were all allocated more or less equitably to the seven districts. The meeting was heated at times. The Chairman said at one point, 'I'm locking the door and no one leaves until each of these sixteen residents is assigned to a district.'

Resolving the plight of the other residents remaining on the non-allocated list was much easier. Districts were informed when one of their residents in the hospital died, and were then requested to select a resident to replace their own from this list. This worked reasonably well and the last residents were taken off the non-allocated list during the last quarter of 1987. Although these two approaches resolved the problem of the districts and the hospital, it was harder on residents who felt as if no plans were being made for them until the last moment before closure.

Slippage

As time progressed, the task force reports began to show that slippage was occurring. The target date for closure was March 1988. At the end of 1985, 50 places had slipped beyond the deadline, and by May 1987 this had increased to 75 and by July 1987 to 100. In fact, on 31 March 1988 there were 118 residents still in the hospital. Sufficient places had been found but they would not be ready on time.

Various factors accounted for this slippage. There was a general problem with building contractors in the south-east because of the high level of private house building/conversion, resulting from the boom in house prices. Building firms were not hungry for work. They were overstretched, and there was little that could be done to speed work up. Housing associations were also overstretched in some cases. The Darenth Park Project applied considerable pressure for the development of a large number of schemes at a more rapid pace than they had been used to. In almost all districts some schemes fell through because of the rapid rise in house prices and the fact that District Valuer's valuations did not keep pace. This meant that other houses had to be found and the process had to begin all over again. Some districts began to experience difficulties recruiting staff, and in particular experienced or qualified staff. This caused the delay of several projects.

None of this was the fault of the Region. Nevertheless, some part of the delay probably was, for it relaxed too early. In 1987 and 1988 it seemed that the part the Region could play had come to an end. The mental handicap co-ordinator became more intensively involved in the production of a strategy for the wider development of mental health services. His work with the Darenth Park Project was in part delegated to others who, while familiar with the issues, lacked his overall view of the project. Other participants, not connected to the project, began to intervene at regional and district levels on particular planning issues, and these activities tended to divert attention from the primary goal of reaching the target date. There was nobody with sufficient authority to stop this from happening. The hard work was thought to be over too soon.

The delays in seeing through the replacement projects seriously impacted on the hospital. Because fewer people were leaving Darenth Park, more staff had to be retained, which subsequently meant that more staff had to be redeployed in a shorter period of time. It also meant that more residents would be discharged in the following year, thereby creating more work for the staff who had to prepare them for it in a shorter period of time. Furthermore, more wards and services had to remain open, thereby reducing the revenue saved. At a time when the pace of the project should have quickened, it actually slowed.

Last minute arrangements

The need for contingency plans in case of slippage was first raised at the May 1987 meeting of the Steering Group. It was then thought that 76 residents would remain in Darenth Park on 31 March 1988 when the hospital ought to be closing. Most of these residents were the responsibility of two districts, Greenwich and West Lambeth, who were requested to come up with contingency plans for them. By the time of the July meeting, the number of residents remaining in Darenth Park at the end of March 1988 had increased to 100 and a third district, Camberwell, was now asked to produce contingency plans.

West Lambeth found it fairly easy to solve the problems of its two groups of residents whose homes would not be ready on time and, as a result, all its residents were transferred from the hospital by the beginning of July. The situation for Greenwich, however, was more complicated. Its contingency plan was to make accommodation available at Goldie Leigh Hospital until each resident's permanent home was ready. This was dependent on other districts taking their remaining residents out of Goldie Leigh. As it happened, Bexley was not able to transfer its 13 residents until the end of August 1988. For Greenwich, this meant there was no space available for the last of their residents to leave Darenth Park when it closed. Camberwell, too, had problems: it was able to rent a house for one group of residents until their intended home was available later in the year, but recruitment problems meant that one home at Bowly Close opened late. A major problem for the district was that it had not made adequate plans for those individuals whose behaviour made it difficult for them to live in close proximity to others. Several of their residents were eventually discharged to a private psychiatric hospital until the district could make adequate provision.

By the time of the May 1988 meeting of the Steering Group, there were still 104 residents in Darenth Park, of whom 24 had confirmed discharge dates. A review of the districts' plans showed that 43 residents would remain in the hospital after 30 June, living in three wards, with the majority of them coming from Greenwich and Camberwell. The hospital had about 14 qualified nursing staff left, who could not adequately cope with the rapid exodus of residents in a very short space of time. Dartford and Gravesham Health Authority was eager to close the hospital and for things not to drag on. There would always be a reason for someone to stay on for another few weeks and the districts had to be forced to take responsibility for their residents. But the hospital manager, and most officers involved in the project, accepted that after all their hard work they did not want the project to end badly. It would have been unfair to residents to have unnecessary moves forced upon them just to keep to a deadline. Therefore, the Steering Group agreed that the hospital could stay open until mid-August, depending on the availability of properties and staff.

As the new deadline approached it became clear that, even then, not everyone would have left the hospital. Those districts still having residents in Darenth Park, i.e. Greenwich and Camberwell, could do little more themselves. It was left to Dartford District to cope. An unused ward at Stone House Hospital, a mental illness hospital, was opened for 12 residents. Temporary use was also made of two houses bought but not yet needed by the

Mental Illness Unit. This allowed the last 20 residents to be discharged from Darenth Park on 12 August 1988.

On 8 September, the sixty-seventh and final meeting of the Darenth Park Steering Group was held, and the group disbanded.

CHAPTER 4

New style planning: the changing role of the region

In Chapter 3 we gave a brief narrative account of the long and complex story of the closure of Darenth Park Hospital, so that readers could keep their bearings in the more detailed analysis that follows. In this chapter, we look in particular at the Region's role in seeking the closure and ask why did they embark on the venture, how did they set about the task, and why did it take so long? In answering these questions we hope to draw lessons that may be of relevance to other health authorities. The analysis also shows that public bureaucracies are neither purely impersonal machines nor are they incapable of adapting to failure and learning new tricks. It is fashionable to see public bodies in a negative light, and to claim that market institutions are the only ones capable of adapting to their environment. This is the story of a public bureaucracy which did, in fact, adapt to its environment, and successfully achieved change.

Why close?

In Chapter 1 we discussed some of the academic theories that have been advanced to explain deinstitutionalization and the forces that lie behind it. How far do these theories find support in the case of Darenth Park?

A study of the South East Metropolitan Hospital Board's records for the period from 1964 to 1974 suggests that concern about the long-stay hospitals in its area had been present for a long time. It was a recurrent worry of the Region's officers without the issue ever publicly surfacing. Plans to modernize Darenth Park had been part of the national hospital plan (Ministry of Health, Cmnd. 1604) in 1962, plans which the Region had submitted and which had been approved by government. In 1964 the report on hospital modernization in the Region had already suggested that the buildings at Darenth Park should ideally be abandoned. It was recognized that the full replacement of the hospital by one of a similar size would be a vast and expensive undertaking, and would recreate the problems associated with large institutions – staffing, management and isolation. Yet the hospital did provide much of the Region's mental handicap facilities and there was a growing demand for such care which local authorities were not providing. Modernization of the hospital and extra facilities in smaller units seemed the only economically feasible way forward.

Difficulties in staff recruitment were also part of Darenth Park's problem as the wider literature in Chapter 1 suggests. A Regional Hospital Board Working Party studied ways of improving mental handicap provision before 1970 and recommended increasing the levels of nursing and domestic staff by at least 250. It was accepted, however, that the major problem was recruiting staff, not finding the extra money.

So far, then, the Darenth Park situation fits the classic accounts of logistical problems faced by large institutions (reviewed in Chapter 1). They were exacerbated by the hospital being in an area of high incomes and chronic labour shortages. However, these long-term economic problems were not enough to prompt closure, and they had been in existence for at least a generation. The economic attraction of selling the site is also vividly exemplified by the saga of the Blue Circle bid. It stimulated the Region to a flurry of activity, and clearly the potential value of the site was always a background factor. The significance of this should not be overestimated. The Blue Circle bid was also a trigger for planning activity, as the intention did not fade when the County Council refused planning permission. Moreover, though the large site was valuable, just how valuable it was depended on another agency, the planning authority, and it was in doubt. The interests that the planning authority represented, e.g. those of local residents, were quite different from the interests of the NHS. Moreover, though the site was potentially valuable, the same economic forces which were pushing up its value were also making other sites expensive and, therefore, very difficult to acquire. It is thus simplistic to suggest that hospital closure was merely a way of cashing in on a valuable site. If we are to understand the Region's motivation we have to dig beneath these superficial explanations.

It is quite clear from the Region's records that had it not been for the Ely scandal (see Chapter 1), its plans for 'upgrading' Darenth Park would simply have gone ahead. Ely had both an impact on national priorities and on the perceptions of officers. The pressures from central government, especially in the form of the Hospital Advisory Service, were important. They did not tell the Region anything it did not know; indeed, the senior medical officer was already considering what should be done with mental handicap services in the Region. However, outside reinforcement of such efforts introduced a new element into the situation, as did the sobering lesson of what could happen if a national scandal were to break, as at Ely.

The Hospital Advisory Service (HAS), as it was then called, paid its first visit to the hospital in February 1970, and made a shorter visit in October of the same year. Many of its critical comments related to the quality of management at the hospital – poor communication among professional groups at senior management level, between nursing administration and ward staff, and between senior management and all other staff at the hospital: 'On arrival the team felt that they had arrived at a house in the middle of a family quarrel.' Interdisciplinary work at all levels needed to be strengthened and medical staff responsibilities reorganized so that each consultant had his own ward which would deal with all types of patients coming from specific local authorities. The second visit, while noting some improvements – particularly an upgrading programme – still pointed to management difficulties as the principal factor behind the lack of an effective provision of services. After visiting other mental handicap units in the Region, a special report was produced by HAS's director which indicated:

1 The need to develop small units throughout the region so that the two large hospitals would not have to cater for patients from the whole region.
2 The importance of the Region's three teaching hospitals becoming involved in mental handicap provision.
3 Links between local authorities and the hospitals needed to be created.

Regarding Darenth Park, the report commented: 'it has such singularly ugly, ill-equipped and badly designed buildings that consideration should be given to its eventual total replacement' (20 April 1970). In the first half of 1972 Darenth Park had a third visit from the Hospital Advisory Service. The team focused on what it considered to be the gross under-financing of the hospital and its staffing situation. It claimed that major capital investment was needed for ward upgrading, catering facilities and support services. There were major staff shortages among domestics and nurses for whom an immediate recruitment campaign should be conducted. The organization of the medical staff was still a concern, and the children's ward was criticized for being too small and for being built in the wrong location.

The Region took all of these criticisms seriously. The parallels with the McDonagh model that we mentioned in Chapter 1 are therefore close. Public scandal and moral outrage about the conditions in mental handicap hospitals and the pressure of a quasi-national inspectorate were not confined to Victorian England. These factors interact with the more prosaic ones of a labour shortage, costs and people's fear of professional disgrace, but to ignore them misses a crucial element in the nature of social policy. So, too, does an emphasis on institutional factors which ignore personalities. We return to this again at the end of this chapter, but here it is important to note the decisive role played by the chairman of the authority at the time. He insisted that action ought to be taken, and that a large capital programme should be embarked upon over the next 10 years even though other projects might have to be delayed. The chairman's background may help us to understand that commitment. Prior to becoming regional chairman he had been chairman for many years of a mental illness hospital and gained an intimate understanding of the problems of long-stay institutions.

A regional advisory team of officers was appointed after the visit of HAS. It estimated that it should be possible to run down Darenth Park from 1550 residents in 1969 to about 800 residents by 1980, simply taking into account existing discharge and death rates if no further residents were admitted. This would roughly match the *Better Services* (DHSS, 1971) target of halving the hospital population by 1980, and matching their norms for provision in the districts concerned. However, when the Regional Hospital Board met in January 1973, it felt that 'the goal now should be to abandon the Darenth Park buildings at the earliest possible date', and it agreed with the chairman that 'the Darenth Park problem was so serious as to warrant an attempt to deal with it in a timescale of ten years' (Minute 61 of the RHB meeting, January 1973). Special capital allocation from the DHSS was to be sought. However, it was not forthcoming and, in the event, closure was to take 15 years, as we saw in Chapter 3. The first 10 years were marked by delays and frustration, the last 5 by much more rapid action. Why was this so? In seeking to answer this question we learn something about the nature of policy implementation and theories of planning.

Why so long?

A detailed account of the frustrations of the first 10 years of Darenth Park's closure is contained in our interim report (Korman and Glennerster, 1985). Here we pick out the major lessons that were learned. The new South East Thames Regional Health Authority, which had just taken over responsibility for hospital capital building in 1974, was also responsible for overall co-ordination of health service provision in the Region following reorganization. It was responsible for prompting area and district health authorities to produce long-term plans, not just for the acute hospitals but for each of the priority client groups. Not least among these groups were people with a mental handicap. It had, as we saw in Chapter 2, clear central guidance on the desirable national norms for provision. It was also under a statutory duty to collaborate with local authorities in providing services for groups like the mentally handicapped.

The Region's officers thus began by following the classical, rational, strategic co-ordinator approach to planning (Glennerster *et al.*, 1983; Challis *et al.*, 1988). A set of planning targets produced by central government formed the basis of the Region's planning advice to its areas and districts. Complementary services were to be provided by local authorities. By sitting down together, it would be possible for representatives of the local authorities, the districts and the Region to produce an acceptable blueprint to which all parties could agree and work. With a joint plan thus agreed, the separate parties would be assigned their different tasks. By appointing representatives of the local authorities, districts and the Region to the Darenth Park Steering Group, it would ensure that all parties kept to the timetable and would resolve any difficulties that occurred.

This procedure assumed agreement on the ultimate goal, the ability to reach a compromise and the means of achieving it, and a degree of good will produced by a common commitment to improve services for mentally handicapped people. Experience was to show how naive these assumptions were.

The limitations of the central rationalist approach

Divergent interests

Even within the regional health authority itself, there were those who were concerned with the general policy of developing services for the mentally handicapped and those who had a special responsibility and interest in the closure of Darenth Park. To a great extent the two groups worked independently, one producing a plan for the mentally handicapped for the Region as a whole, the other working towards the closure of Darenth Park. At the local level, local voluntary organizations, community health councils and district health care planning teams were much more concerned about the paucity of local services for the mentally handicapped already living in the community. While discussion within the Steering Group was concerned with the progress of plans for replacement units for the Darenth Park residents, discussions in the districts largely concerned the development of community services for the general population. Priorities for action were quite different. Moreover, the kinds of new facilities suggested by the Region fitted into its replacement needs, not those of local communities. Large units made transfer from the hospital easier but were not necessarily appropriate to the long-term needs of the new generation of mentally handicapped people in each of the communities. They were, moreover, increasingly unacceptable to families with mentally handicapped children. This is where the divergent interests of local communities and the changing philosophies of care came together.

Divergent models of care

Using the norms detailed in *Better Services* (DHSS, 1971), the Region calculated that the largest number of places each district would require would be 184. This was comfortably below the maximum size of unit which the DHSS had recommended. The Region's planners, therefore, advocated that each district should provide on one site sufficient places for all of its mentally handicapped. This would involve a site of perhaps 10–16 acres each. The preference was for new buildings, or conversions (e.g. teacher training colleges) if new sites could not be found. This would simplify the problems of building design, planning and the transfer of residents from hospital. The sheer practical problems of locating such sites were soon recognized, but as area health authorities and local groups responded to these plans it became clear that such large concentrations of handicapped people and the kind of institutions that would result were unacceptable locally, and thus a compromise was put forward by the Region. Its suggestion was for a residential centre for 72 of the most severely handicapped, to consist of both houses and flats, each of which would accommodate about six people. Also to be made available on the same site were a day centre, available to people from the community as well as residents, and a base for the community mental handicap team and for the management of the mental handicap services in the district. Hostels in the community were to cater for 24 residents each, again sub-divided into groups of six. These guidelines were further amended after local consultation to include reference to local authority provision, and for the first time to the possible provision of group homes where several people could live in traditional housing.

Despite the willingness of the Region to compromise and produce new guidelines, they could not satisfy everyone. Indeed, they probably did not satisfy anyone fully. Opinions about appropriate kinds of care for mentally handicapped people were changing fast. Preferred local models ranged from those who wished to see almost complete reliance on the use of the traditional housing, to much more traditional modes. Seeking to get everybody to conform to a single norm, albeit a flexible one, meant that every district felt a certain resentment.

Perverse financial incentives

From the beginnings of the NHS itself, there had been a perverse financial incentive built in. If the NHS provided hospital facilities for the mentally handicapped, the central Exchequer, not the local ratepayers, footed the bill. Now the NHS hoped local authorities could be persuaded to foot more of the bill, providing support facilities, day centres, training centres, as well as the care of the less handicapped who were now in Darenth Park. In addition, local authorities were to provide services for families whose children could not now be admitted to Darenth Park. In parallel with this, central government was beginning to cut back the financial support it was giving to local authorities after the 1976 economic crisis. In these circumstances, it was not surprising that local authorities essentially refused to collaborate unless they were paid to do so. Under the rules as they existed before 1983, as we saw in Chapter 2, this was not possible.

No incentives for cooperation

Shortly before the Darenth Park Steering Group was set up, the local authorities were approached about their involvement, and more specifically the possibility of their accepting responsibility for those patients who did not require hospital care, and were therefore inappropriately placed at Darenth Park. Their response, several months later, was to request funds to undertake an assessment of each resident at the hospital to determine what alternative placement would be satisfactory. The intention was to appoint a team consisting of a social worker for each local authority, a project leader and a clerical assistant, the cost of which was estimated at £80 000 per annum for two years. The directors of social services stated that the cost of employing the social workers to carry out such an assessment and to assist in the planned movement of patients would have to be borne wholly by the NHS. This was their attitude throughout the project. They argued that community care could not entail that transfer of responsibilities without the transfer of resources. In 1978, the regional team of officers did approve £50 000 per annum for two years for an assessment team, to be charged against the Region's joint finance allocation. However, the directors of social services were adamant that the NHS bear the full cost. They stated that they would withdraw from the Steering Group and from cooperation at regional and area levels if this sum of money was not forthcoming. In light of this, the regional team of officers and the RHA reconsidered, and in November 1978 agreed to the full sum.

The results of the pilot social work assessment of 123 residents was discussed at a meeting of the Steering Group in 1980, attended by all the directors of social services in the catchment area. The assessment showed that about 30% of the residents could immediately be considered suitable for local authority or voluntary organization care. Local authorities said they expected the NHS to make available capital and revenue funds to provide for this care. In 1981, one of the local authorities, Southwark, found a house that was suitable for conversion into a small hostel able to accommodate 10 people. The authority said it was willing to use it for residents from Darenth Park, but this project would be additional to the social services departments' plans and required finance from the health authority to pay for it. The NHS claimed that joint finance was the only mechanism available to transfer funds to the local authority, and could therefore give no support. The local authority would accept 100% revenue funding for seven years. The area health authority felt unable to agree to this because it would take too high a proportion of the joint finance allocation for many years to come. The Region, also involved in these discussions, was unwilling to increase the area health authority's joint finance allocation to take account of this additional project on the grounds that it would be unfair to other districts in the region. A series of meetings between area, region and local authority officers was unable to resolve the problem, and so a Regional Health Authority members' meeting was held in February 1982. When the RHA said they were unable to transfer additional funds for this project, the local authority members and officers withdrew from the meeting and from collaboration at regional level. They did not return until the Region produced the mental handicap funding policy to which we return later.

No regional sanctions, no local goodwill

Though the Region was able to advise and recommend targets and guidelines, it could not actually either plan or deliver local services, only the districts could do that. In between was a second tier of planning authorities, the area health authorities. Though they wanted to press ahead with the planning process, they were more interested in developing local services rather than

solving the Region's problems. There was no procedure such as accountability reviews that enabled the Region to bring sanctions to bear on either
areas or districts. The area tier merely confused the lines of accountability and
made it difficult for the Region to communicate with the districts. Furthermore, the districts which were to provide the facilities were in the main in
London, and were losing resources because of the application of the RAWP
formula to the Region. The Region, because of population movements, was
withdrawing funds from London, which did not enamour it to either area or
district members.

Effective local sanctions

If the Region could not impose sanctions on districts or local authorities for
failing to plan or develop alternative services, local authorities and local
groups did have effective blocking power over the Region's plans. They could
hold up planning permission for new sites or conversions. In one district, the
purchase of a site was delayed by over two years because of hostility by
certain pressure groups to a plan for a residential centre. Two other districts
effectively dropped out of the Darenth Park Project and developed their own
district plans. A fourth district took three years to reach agreement with its
local authority because key figures from both sides were not happy with the
plan for the main site.

   Thus, if we take all of these factors together it is not surprising that so little
was achieved in the period up to 1983. They illustrate the weakness of the
original strategic co-ordinator theory of planning. What we see reflected here
is what Lindblom (1965) calls 'partisan mutual adjustment'. By this he means
that separate organizations with very different interests reach accommo-
dations with one another by a variety of competitive strategies. In so far as the
Region was able to make progress, it did so by what Lindblom calls
'disjointed incrementalism'. By this he means a process of continuous
problem solving. The Region would see an opportunity to develop a
particular site or to reach agreement with a particular organization, would
seek to advance that particular solution at that particular time, and then as
another problem arose its officers would seek to resolve that. However, this
was not a method that produced rapid or sustained progress towards the goal
of closing Darenth Park within the alloted time-scale. It needed a new set of
external pressures, a new set of actors and new legal powers to break the
log-jam. Above all, Regional officers learned to adapt their style of planning
and management. 'Institutional learning' took place.

New mechanisms to manage change

The Region's officers evolved several important changes in the approach
which we mentioned briefly in the previous chapter.

Mobilizing consent and establishing a network of communication

The Steering Group was used to greater effect not only as a formal body but to legitimate contacts between key local actors. The Darenth Park Steering Group represented the local health authorities (after 1982, district health authorities), the hospital, social services departments in the catchment area and regional officers most deeply involved in the project. The Steering Group was unique in so far as the project was unique – it took the Darenth Park Replacement Project out of the annual planning system and gave priority to developed schemes in the capital programme. It focused the attention of senior officers – in the Region, in areas and later districts, and in local authorities – on the range of issues to be tackled to complete the project. It enabled links to be made between the key actors in the different authorities which other studies on inter-corporate planning suggest is important (Friend *et al.*, 1974). By taking Darenth Park out of the annual planning system, it also bypassed those officers who did not agree that such priority should be given to closing the hospital. It should not be assumed that regional officers presented a monolithic outlook on particular issues, and the development of mental handicap services was no exception. As we have observed, some regional officers favoured an approach which gave priority to developing community services first to prevent further admissions to hospitals. By creating a 'planning system' just for the Darenth Park Project, this confrontation was avoided.

A new approach to capital planning

The decision to move to traditional housing enabled capital planning decisions to be decentralized. Instead of making their way through a complex system of capital approval and individual project cost control, small schemes could be approved if they fell within an average bed space cost limit. Individual housing associations and local officers had scope to find their own solutions. In order to achieve this change it was necessary for the new mental handicap planning co-ordinator to overcome resistance from parts of the regional bureaucracy who were opposed. The regional works department had an obvious interest in maintaining the works programme of purpose-built units. The treasurer's department was initially not happy about handing over NHS funds to other organizations, or providing services for others to run. Working with districts and housing associations would change the basis of the Region's existing methods of work and working relationships; in particular, it represented a loss of control over projects and of control over details.

A new financial incentive structure

A major innovation was the decision to change the funding policy in such a way as to give financial incentives to districts and other organizations to cooperate. This was to prove a decisive breakthrough. The Region's problem was simple: it had begun the Darenth Park Project under the old system of capital planning, which allocated additional revenue to districts to meet the cost of running new premises – 'revenue consequences of capital schemes' (RCCS). By 1982, the rules of capital funding had changed – RCCS was no longer available. Districts were now being required to show how they would be able to meet the revenue costs of new schemes themselves as part of the Capricode planning system. More importantly, the Region no longer had new growth funds each year to use in this way. The RAWP system of allocation of funds to regions was beginning to be applied more rigorously. The Region had been informed by the DHSS that it could effectively expect to have no new growth funds for the next few years. The districts in the Darenth Park Project area were at the inner-London end of the Region, and in some cases were well over their RAWP targets. Even if the Region had funds available, it would have been reluctant to channel them to these districts, because it would make their RAWP position worse, and it would limit its capacity to reallocate revenue to other parts of the Region.

On the other hand, from the start of the project, districts had made it plain to the Region that they could not fund new mental handicap services from their existing resources. Districts, too, were coming under tighter cash constraints, and claimed they were rationalizing services to stay within cash limits. There was nothing spare to fund new services. Without the Region being able to transfer funds to them, districts would refuse to open new facilities.

It was this log-jam which the new funding proposals broke. At the end of 1982, the regional treasurer produced a new funding policy which capitalized on some of the ideas put forward in the government's consultative paper *Care in the Community* (DHSS, 1981b). The first step was to calculate what it would cost to keep residents in hospital. The treasurer used an estimate of the numbers who would remain in hospital by 1992 if there were no change in the pattern of discharge. By using a 1992 projection, deaths and discharges over this 10-year period would reduce the inpatient population, and therefore increase the cost per resident. That figure formed the basis for the 'dowry'. Each resident taken out of hospital by any district in the Region would receive a standard annual income which became known as the dowry system. This represented a revenue transfer to districts in perpetuity, regardless of the initial degree of handicap of the resident.

Working the funding policy in this way produced several advantages. First, it eliminated detailed negotiations between the districts and the Region. If the per capita revenue was the same, it eliminated drawn-out negotiations on the level of capacity of each resident. The funding policy created some degree of certainty for districts. They now knew how much they could expect to receive from the Region depending on how many residents they took. Next, the funding policy, by channelling inpatient revenue to districts, could be seen as giving districts new funds without reducing the long-term funds available in the Region. Thirdly, as part of the funding policy, the Region removed the mental handicap funding from the general RAWP system, and treated it separately. This allowed funds to be given to districts for new mental handicap services without worsening their overall RAWP position. Finally, Regional officers were able to show that the amount received by almost every district for the total number of dowries it was likely to receive would still leave districts below the figure implied in the RAWP formula. Districts would still need to find additional funds for mental handicap services. Up to that stage, no one really had any idea what was an 'adequate' amount of funds for mental handicap services.

The way the funding policy operated also contributed to the capacity of the Region to devolve responsibility to districts. Each resident came with a dowry, regardless of the type of facility he or she would be living in. The funding policy was not tied to particular types of developments. It therefore allowed districts to make local provision in line with local wishes, without being driven by a regionally agreed policy.

The funding policy aimed to produce fairly simple and clear principles which avoided the Region becoming involved in detailed negotiations with districts. It had several guidelines:

1 It applied only to patients resident in the named hospitals before April 1983. Admissions after that time were subject to negotiation between the DHAs involved.
2 Districts would receive the standard amount as an addition to their cash limit (pro-rata in the year of transfer depending on the date of the move, and a full annual amount thereafter).
3 Districts could negotiate with local authorities, private or voluntary organizations if there were clinical or social reasons why a resident would benefit more from care provided by another organization. The charges made for such services could be above or below the standard dowry, depending on the costs of care and the availability of other sources of funding.
4 Funding was available to other organizations as long as they went on providing a similar service. For existing private or voluntary organization services, this usually meant the life of the resident. If services were specifically created for the Darenth Park residents by a local voluntary organization or a social services department, funding would continue as long as the project continued to care for people who otherwise might have required health service provision. In practice, this has meant simply providing a continuing service for the same client group. The important point was that funding was tied to a project, not named individuals.

The weakness of the funding policy was that the sum offered was not enough to pay for all services required locally by individuals. It represented a share of all services theoretically received at the hospital – residential and day care, paramedical and medical support, nurse training, and administrative overheads. Regional officers admitted that it would not be enough to cover full care in the community but that there was no other source of funds within the Region. The Region did contribute an additional £1 million towards the cost of special needs services (see below), but this was for the whole of the region, not solely the Darenth Park districts.

Regional officers, the Regional Treasurer in particular, recognized that the districts would still need to find additional revenue for services from their general allocation. This became increasingly difficult as cash limits became tighter. Several districts delayed opening new facilities while they tried to get additional funding from the Region, with varying degrees of success. In one district, a pre-election bonus helped to bail out the mental handicap programme which had been brought to a stop by the district management board on the grounds it could not afford to provide the additional money.

Another difficulty was the date at which the transfer of funds began. The Region was to advance dowries up to three months before a resident was discharged, to enable staff to be appointed in advance and start working with the residents before they moved. However, this was simply an advance on the money due to the district in that financial year: the total remained the same. Inevitably, this caused the districts difficulty.

That in its turn reflected a major problem that the Region faced, i.e. its inability to get money out of the hospitals that were losing residents fast enough. The dowry for each resident was the same regardless of which hospital they came from. Obviously, different hospitals had different running costs, so the amount withdrawn had to relate to that hospital's average inpatient expenditure; otherwise, some hospitals would lose all their funding before all residents left, and others would have lost all residents while still having funds available. In 1981–2, the average inpatient costs varied from £4834 to £13 500.

In addition to the hospitals' fixed costs, plant and heating, many key staff remained even if marginal costs were falling. Marginal costs were less than average costs. Fixed overheads decreased only when whole wards or blocks were closed, not simply when one or two residents left. Therefore, the Region and hospitals negotiated on an annual basis how much could be withdrawn and, naturally, each hospital argued that it could not return to the full average cost assumed in the funding policy. The funding policy thus went into 'debt' from about the fourth year, borrowing from other regional funds, such as the mental illness funding policy, to cover this 'bridging' finance.

Nor did the funding policy make any allowance for putting extra funds into the hospitals during the run-down period. In the case of Darenth Park this led to a decline in some aspects of the physical environment and its inability to recruit staff. These are also aspects of the policy from which other regions may learn.

Providing leadership

It is still somewhat unusual in the NHS to find an officer willing to step out of 'standard operating procedures' and openly take a leadership role on a controversial issue. Without the regional nursing officer (now director of personnel and manpower planning) who did this, the Darenth Park Project would not have succeeded.

It was the regional nursing officer (RNO) who gave evidence to the Public Enquiry on the sale of Darenth Park to Blue Circle, and who two months later chaired the Darenth Park Steering Group. It was also the RNO who secured the backing of the chairman of the RHA and of RHA members making the closure of Darenth Park a regional priority. Over the 10 years, she gave the project a sense of continuity, belying the many changes which took place in the NHS during this time. It was also the RNO who took it upon herself to see that all obstacles were overcome – negotiating with colleagues at the regional level to bend the rules to get what was needed for the closure of Darenth Park. Before general management came in, the RNO acted like a manager.

That was not enough however. More officers needed to meet regularly to chase the progress of the multiple parts of the project and find solutions to practical problems as they arose.

When the Darenth Park Project began, there were four regional officers involved; however, the involvement of each was limited. It was simply something additional to their existing responsibilities. The result of this situation was that issues tended to get lost in between meetings of the Steering Group, not followed up or not resolved. Moreover, because support from the district and regional officers not involved in the project was tenuous, any issue raised which seemed to challenge the viability of the project or its basic planning philosophy made the regional officers react very strongly. This lack of support for the project made any criticism or deviation seem threatening, and therefore unacceptable.

One of the ways in which this situation was overcome was to bring together a group of people who *were* committed to the Darenth Park Project: the prime concern of both the regional staff training co-ordinator and the mental handicap planning co-ordinator was with Darenth Park; the start of the mental handicap funding policy linked in the treasurer's department on a more regular basis; a quantity surveyor was drawn in to keep an overview of some of the problems arising with several regional schemes; and the public relations department became more actively involved with publicity material for the opening of the residential centres.

In 1984, a formal regional task force was created, initially to speed up the new housing programme. The task force gradually expanded its remit to include all the other officers not directly involved with housing as mentioned above. They took up any problem which threatened to sidetrack progress on the closure programme.

The group was primarily problem-oriented. It had pre-Steering Group discussions of agendas to identify what issues were likely to come up, and how these were to be handled. It tried to ensure that all officers likely to be in contact with the districts were giving out the same message. Their members also leant support to each other, as they could understand the difficulties each faced in their respective tasks. The task force overcame the initial sense of isolation, felt by the regional officers who began the project. Through the task force, and through the sense of determination and strength it gave its members, regional officers were able to take a much more active role in keeping districts moving towards closure. Regional officers often needed to take on a brokerage role between districts, not necessarily pushing its own solution but seeing that districts reached *some* agreement. For example, this was necessary in the case of Greenwich and the other districts using Goldie Leigh Hospital, and Lewisham and North Southwark and Bromley in relation to Grove Park.

In brief

1 We have argued that the generalized accounts of deinstitutionalization which we referred to in Chapter 1 do find echoes in the history of Darenth Park. The practical and economic pressures for the closure were present, but they had been present for a long time. The actual story is more complex. The precipitating factors which made closure a feasible option were several: the scandal associated with Ely and central government pressure for action; external inspection of the conditions that existed at Darenth Park; the fear of scandal that would reflect on the Region's officers; the genuine concern by regional officers and the regional chairman of public concern; and the possible windfall that would follow from the sale of the site. The new ideological pressure behind normalization was also a contributory factor. In the early stages this challenged accepted views and made progress more difficult. In the long run, however, because it justified the unlocking of additional social security funding and made the acquisition of traditional housing more likely, it won practical support from managers.

2 The original model of central planning failed, but sustained regional interest and continuous pressure on the districts to produce results was important. So too was the setting of a definite deadline for closure. To be effective, however, this central pressure had to be combined with the freedom of districts to produce their own solutions. The new model is very similar to the principles of 'tight and loose management' followed by some of the most successful private corporations (Peters and Waterman, 1982). A strong lead is coupled with maximum devolution of managerial responsibility.

3 Pressure for results would have got nowhere without a financial regime which gave incentives to districts and other agencies to provide new places. Bureaucracies need an appropriate incentive structure to respond to national policy. This is now much more widely accepted, but in the early days of the Darenth Park Project it was not. Those involved had to learn those lessons for themselves and to invent new incentive structures. This lesson was learned and the new funding mechanisms operated to great effect. In short, public servants can be innovative and public bureaucracies can adapt if they are given the freedom to do so.

CHAPTER 5

Getting services ready for people

The story up to 1982

As we have already seen, the original intention was that the task of preparing services for Darenth Park residents would be a joint enterprise between the local authorities in the catchment area and the NHS. For reasons we have already discussed, this never materialized. The local authorities were only prepared to participate if they were given the financial resources to do so; however, this was not legally possible in the early stages of the project. There was also a basic reluctance on the part of NHS officers to hand over 'their' resources to another organization over whom they had no control. As the economics of bureaucracies suggests to us (Niskanen, 1971; Mueller, 1979), public servants gain power, prestige, satisfaction and, more arguably, income if they manage larger organizations with larger budgets. Put in these crude terms the theory is simplistic (Dunleavy, 1987). There are also costs to managing a large organization, e.g. stress and the loss of direct control. Even so, our discussions with health managers over the long life of the project suggests that given the financial resources at their disposal, they would rather have had the satisfaction of managing the reprovision task themselves, or to do so with organizations from whom they could buy services direct rather than working with another much more political, unpredictable agency over whom they had little control. The management styles of local authorities and the NHS began to diverge more after the coming of general management. The new unit general managers had clear management tasks and more independence. They were not worried by what their political bosses might say, and they could afford to be experimental. At the same time, the local authorities were becoming more political. Finally, because the local authorities had been out of the planning process for so long the die was cast by 1983. The habit of collaboration had not been cultivated. The NHS had learned to go its own unilateral way without the time-consuming task of joint action and detailed consultation. Thus even when the financial rules of the game changed in 1983, the health districts who had become the prime agencies in reprovision continued to be so. We discuss what collaboration there was in Chapter 7, but the first legacy of the period prior to 1983 was that the tasks of reprovision fell to the district health authorities.

The new funding policy and the Region's determination to close the hospital at a set date had helped to solve the second legacy of the period before 1983 – districts' primary concern with developing services for their existing population, not the Darenth Park residents. The real urgency to find places by 1988 was combined with the fact that the 'dowries' that came with the residents of Darenth Park were virtually the only growth money districts were receiving.

The Region's officers became much more relaxed about accepting schemes which involved the use of ordinary housing, as we saw in Chapter 4. More than that, they organized workshops and conferences to spread the gospel. Added to this, the coming of general management introduced a new group of managers to many districts, some of whom came with the conviction that normalization should be the driving force behind reprovision. Others came largely ignorant of the whole field of mental handicap but quickly learned the new gospel. Moreover, these new managers were *service* providers, responsible for planning the new services, not planners pure and simple. All these factors gave a new impetus to districts' activities. Within two years of restructuring, many of the inherited plans had changed.

The new plans

We review each district's progress before discussing some of the general problems and lessons that can be drawn. The account illustrates the range of sheer practical difficulties that arose.

Dartford and Gravesham

A project team had been set up in 1977 to begin planning a replacement unit for Dartford and Gravesham residents in Darenth Park. The design and thinking behind it predated even the Steering Group guidelines. The District's main facility was to be a residential centre – four separate buildings for 24 residents each, divided internally into two separate wings, each with their own bedrooms, day rooms, kitchen and bathrooms. These buildings would be able to accommodate 96 residents. The site chosen was less than ideal as a community facility, as it had a mental illness hospital (to be closed some time during the 1990s) on one side, another long-stay hospital currently used by the district treasurer's department on another side, a housing estate at the rear boundary and a rubbish dump (at some stage due to become a leisure centre) in front. Its main or only advantage was that it was owned by the NHS and had no other buildings on it. A 120-place day centre for use by the residents and other people with a mental handicap from the community was also to be provided on site. The site was to be further shared by a new school for nurse training. This was an excellent example of the way service provision was

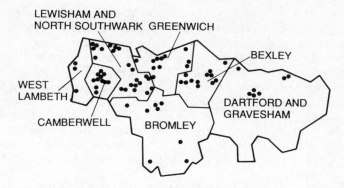

Figure 5.1 Residential facilities for mentally handicapped people, 1988.

being driven by site availability. The character of the service also reflects the stage at which the plans were originally drawn up.

In addition, the District planned a 24-place hostel. Because a site could not be found, four group homes were substituted. Not only did the group homes give some flexibility to a more old-fashioned service model, they also allowed staff to observe the ways in which residents developed and showed their capabilities in more normal settings.

The new residential centre, Archery House, and day centre buildings were handed over in mid-1985. Immediately, the officers who were actually to run the service ran into problems which reflected that insufficient detailed thought had gone into the design stage. It was impossible to furnish the bedrooms fully as planned and cater for wheelchair-bound residents at the same time. It became evident that one bed per room would need to be removed to facilitate wheelchair manoeuvrability. Consequently, the number of places available at the residential centre was reduced from 96 to 80. The District therefore had to create new places elsewhere, and quickly. Furthermore, at about the same time, Dartford and Gravesham was faced with the closure of other smaller local facilities.

It was decided to appoint a project officer to explore suitable private and voluntary sector provision, a post that was to be financed from joint finance money over a period of three years. An experienced social worker was also appointed, whose objective was to find a minimum of 16 places in private, voluntary or family homes. In fact, she was able to find alternative accommodation for more than 30 adults: 12 in private registered homes, 8 in family placement schemes initiated by the social worker, 7 in two maisonnettes rented from the council in the name of the social worker, 2 in flats rented directly by the tenants from the council, and 2 in an unregistered private home.

Most of the residents placed by the social worker came from Archery House. The move proposed represented a further step towards more independent living for the residents. The basis of this successful venture was the way in which the social worker was able to offer reassurance to staff that residents would be well cared for in the new facilities and to make them aware of the potential for greater independence for residents. As a result, the attitudes of the care staff towards the residents changed considerably and an active programme of preparation for more independent living was commenced. It was significant that such a change in attitudes was brought about by someone coming from outside the hospital setting. It was all too easy for staff at Archery House, all of whom had previously worked at Darenth Park, to transfer attitudes across to their new situation. It was also a very good example of what could be achieved by adapting the care manager approach recommended in the Griffiths Report (DHSS, 1988). In effect, that is what this social worker did.

Thus, despite initial difficulties, Dartford and Gravesham was able to provide for all its Darenth Park residents and in a more imaginative way than the original plans would have allowed.

Bromley

The original plans for Bromley included a 72-place residential centre with a day centre and staff accommodation, and three 24-place hostels. In 1983, the District had agreed to abandon the plans for the third hostel and make more intensive use of the first purpose-built facilities it would be getting and of additional beds in an existing hostel for women with a mild mental handicap. In the following year, the District agreed to drop the plans for the second hostel when DHA members, attending the Region's training course on staffed group homes, urged the development of additional group homes.

The original plan was revised. It would use the first purpose-built hostel as a training centre for one intake of residents and then transfer these residents to houses purchased with the capital intended for the second hostel. These houses would be handed over to housing associations and the higher level of social security benefits which the residents would receive would help to improve the overall financial position, while also providing a better service than that offered by another hostel.

The senior mental handicap staff clearly did not feel confident about basing all residential services on small homes. Yet they were well aware of the changes taking place in professional values. They wanted to ensure that the services they provided did not prevent or limit the development of individuals. Therefore, they decided to modify their plans for both the kind of care and the kind of staff employed at the residential centre and in the hostels. They proposed to have only care staff who would be responsible for all necessary home-making functions. Residents would participate in these activities and receive 'reward' money. At the residential centre, various centralized services were to be dropped (e.g. laundry and catering), and moved to the individual houses as well. In the day centre, plans were modified to allow more active participation by the residents in all the services provided there.

Bexley

Bexley's original plan was to use 80 places at Goldie Leigh Hospital on a temporary basis until a large enough site for a residential centre became available in the borough. A 24-place hostel, located opposite the district administrative headquarters, was already in the Region's capital programme.

During 1983, two new staff were appointed, both of whom had previously worked for Camberwell Health Authority, and who favoured a new approach. They both suggested a greater use of traditional housing in Bexley, and were supported by the Community Health Council (CHC) and Mencap. This move was further strengthened by the health authority's decision to participate in a DHSS-sponsored programme to remove children under 16 from mental handicap hospitals.

The District's early attempts at buying houses in the community had failed, in one case because of sustained opposition from neighbours and the subsequent refusal of planning permission by the Council. In this instance, some district officers wanted to appeal to the Secretary of State. Lack of parking facilities was cited as the reason for planning permission not being granted, though this was obviously spurious. The local authority was embarrassed at having to defend itself for not granting planning permission. In return for DHA officers agreeing to drop the appeal against the Council's refusal to grant planning permission, the Council made another site available and agreed to work with the DHA on other sites to ensure that planning permission was approached in a smoother manner.

The process was eased by the outcome of the negotiations on the distribution of non-catchment residents. As a result, Bexley need only provide accommodation for its 64 catchment residents, rather than the 110 the District thought it would need to accommodate. With 24 places already programmed for the hostel, it made less sense to consider using Goldie Leigh Hospital for a very much smaller number of adults.

A third factor was the attendance of Bexley Health Authority and social services staff at the regional training co-ordinator's course on staffed accommodation. This course helped to build support for the new types of service and provide practical advice which gave staff confidence in their ability to create and manage the group homes and traditional housing.

The outcome was a decision not to use the Goldie Leigh site at all. The remaining 40 places needed by the District would all be in houses bought in the community. By the end of 1985, the District had acquired homes for all but 10 of their residents. Negotiations started with housing associations in October 1985 to take over the houses. At the same time, discussions began about the establishment of a Mental Handicap Consortium to undertake the housing management aspect of these properties. (We discuss the consortium concept at the end of this chapter as it was implemented differently in different districts.)

Greenwich

In 1981, Greenwich opened a 30-place hostel, formerly used as a geriatric convalescent home, for both Greenwich and Bexley residents from Darenth Park. The District's plans in the period immediately after restructuring consisted of a 32-place hostel already in the regional capital programme, and a residential centre on the site of the Royal Herbert, a former military hospital. This development began as a 72-place centre, but by 1982 this had fallen to 48. As detailed previously (see Korman and Glennerster, 1985), these plans were not reached easily. Greenwich Borough, the CHC and some professional staff had urged the health authority to provide services based in small community houses rather than purpose-built facilities. This was overruled by the health authority on the grounds of the need to meet the closure deadline and the lack of evidence yet available that small houses were suitable for all types of residents.

A new director of nursing services in mental handicap was appointed as a result of the 1982 restructuring. Plans continued for the Royal Herbert site until 1985, when District dissatisfaction with the amount of space available within the accommodation reached a stage which made further progress unlikely. The problem was one familiar to all districts in the south-east of England – to keep within the unrealistic cost limits meant building to 70–80% of the required space. This in turn meant that residents in wheelchairs would be difficult to accommodate. District officers wanted to take the problem to the DHSS and make a special case for permission to overspend the limit for the project, but regional officers prevaricated. The Region's position had usually been to urge progress to keep to deadlines. The Borough's planning committee had also refused planning permission for the Royal Herbert site in July 1985, on the overt grounds that members wanted to see the overall plans for the site before approving the plans for part of it. In fact, residents in the area were objecting to the development.

A further problem for the District was that 69 of its residents were still in Darenth Park, but only 48 alternative places had been planned for them. To cover this shortfall, it began discussions with housing associations about using housing stock in the community. Social services officers asked to be part of these discussions, as this was the type of provision they had been urging all along.

Within a year, Greenwich's plans had changed quite radically. The Region had told the District that the Royal Herbert site was no longer available, because it now had hopes of selling it to a supermarket chain. A new Unit General Manager (UGM) was appointed in early 1986 who favoured greater collaboration with social services. Under pressure from the social services department, the District reconsidered its intentions to relocate the purpose-built units on another site and agreed instead to make provision for 43 residents to be transferred to the care of the social services department with full capital and revenue costs. In addition, alternative plans were discussed for a smaller day centre.

At the time of writing, discussions are under way to transfer the District's purpose-built hostel to a housing association and to seek permission to sell the other hostel, rehousing its residents in ordinary houses. Once again, practical factors had forced the District to provide ordinary housing and hostel provision rather than a larger residential centre.

Lewisham and North Southwark

The plans in Lewisham and North Southwark were modified only slightly. The original intention was to pilot a core and cluster development. In 1984, when the District agreed to take a larger number of residents from Darenth Park than it needed to in order to meet its *Better Services* (DHSS, 1971) guidelines (it already had Grove Park Hospital with 160 places), staff agreed to go ahead with the use of ordinary housing throughout the service, dropping the idea of a core and cluster development. The District needed to take only 24 more residents from Darenth Park, although there were 81 catchment residents at the hospital. The District was prepared to take all of these residents, but only if they received funding for them. The Region had previously set a limit on the number of residents transferring to Lewisham and North Southwark whom they would fund. To overcome this problem, a new funding arrangement was negotiated whereby the Region would allow all 81 residents to receive the dowry payment if, when Darenth Park was closed, the District worked towards the closure of Grove Park Hospital whence the Region would recoup its initial outlay by withdrawing funds from the District.

Camberwell Health Authority

Camberwell Health Authority, as King's Health District, had agreed to a 72-place residential centre at Bowley Close, Crystal Palace. The land was a disused part of British Rail Crystal Palace station and, although planning for this development began in 1979, the site was not purchased from the Greater London Council (GLC) until 1984, due in part to local residents' and CHC opposition to the proposed scheme, taken to heart by some GLC councillors.

Once again, thinking within the district changed. A Community and Mental Handicap Services Unit had been created in the 1982 restructuring, and the staff appointed were drawn more towards principles of normalization than towards a more traditional approach to service provision. They had on either side of them (Lewisham and North Southwark, and West Lambeth) two districts whose style of service would be based on housing in the community. Both the assistant unit administrator and the unit administrator attended a Programme Analysis of Service Systems (PASS) workshop and they and several others attended the regional course on staffed housing. A group home for eight residents opened in 1983. Officers selected quite able residents for these two flats, which perhaps gave a somewhat misleading impression that all residents would be able to adapt easily to small homes. A further factor was that, having no existing services, there was no one in the District to speak for an alternative model or to claim advantages for the residential centre. The District's own financial planning showed that the provision of a large number of places in ordinary housing in the community would result in revenue savings to the NHS over the cost of the residential centre.

The outcome was that the District proposed to reduce Bowley Close in size to 42 places, the extra 30 places being provided by community housing. The Region agreed, with the proviso that the additional places in community housing be identified within a year and that planning for 72 places would continue until it was certain that alternative accommodation would be found in time. Due largely to the enthusiasm of the assistant unit administrator working with housing associations, sufficient community places were found within 12 months, and the Region formally agreed to a reduction in the number of residential places in 1985.

West Lambeth

Regional officers used the *Better Services* (DHSS, 1971) norms as the basis for calculating the number of places needed in West Lambeth, but it was scarcely realistic to assume the District would take that number of residents from Darenth Park, as it was known to have about 88 residents at St Lawrence's hospital in the South-West Thames Region. The 1984 agreement required the District to take only 30 residents from Darenth Park. On that basis, the District began to make plans for all accommodation to be in group homes. It realized that, without the dowries, no funds for mental handicap facilities would be available.

Overview

We can see from these individual accounts that 'normalization' proved a godsend to local planners. Local residents objected to large sites for the use by mentally handicapped people and were successful in blocking planning permission. Cost limits were unrealistically low. Ordinary housing and the use of money from the DHSS provided a way out which had a philosophical justification.

It is not surprising that some accommodation was not ready when Darenth Park was closed, considering the number of changes that were made to districts' plans between two and four years before closure.

A difficult adjustment

We have seen that a major change of approach took place regarding the principles that underlay service provision, partly for positive and partly for negative reasons. The districts were to find that normalization was not that easy to achieve. Let us now illustrate some of the more general problems with specific examples.

A *new set of actors*

So far, the primary inter-authority relationships had been between NHS and social services departments of local authorities with planning committees acting as the means by which local residents' sanctions could be exercised. The fact that existing housing was to be used increased the *number* of sites for which permission was required, which brought the housing department into the bargaining process. In Greenwich, the DHA had hoped to purchase three sites from the Borough on which it intended to build or upgrade houses. These sites were to be taken over by housing associations and the care staff in them were to be provided and managed by the social services department. However, there were a few problems. First, the Planning Committee insisted on wheelchair access throughout all houses. Secondly, neighbours objected to the purchase of one house, and therefore a second round of consultations had to be held with them. Managers went to call on them and discussed the issues at length, reassuring them and allaying their fears. Thirdly, a few months after this, the Borough attempted to attach some provisos to the way the land sites were used, in particular whether any part of one site could be sold. The Housing Committee then asked that the sites be revalued by the district valuer because their value had increased since first being valued seven months earlier. The final twist was that the Housing Committee decided to link the sale of these three sites to negotiations about the use of the site of a hospital that had recently closed. In February 1988 the project team aborted all attempts to purchase these sites from the Borough.

The need for good local management and funding commitment

Camberwell exemplifies this well. Because of a prolonged leave of absence, and then resignation, the District lacked a key manager to plan and implement at an early but critical phase, and thus the momentum went out of the project for several years.

There seems to have been a serious lack of commitment on behalf of the District as a whole to the Darenth Park Project. This was expressed in several ways. One was a reluctance to supply sufficient administrative and planning resources to see the project through adequately. Senior officers created no structure to undertake the significant amount of planning support needed before anyone could move out of Darenth Park, and there was considerable reluctance to meet the requests of the unit for additional staff appointments. An equally serious manifestation of the lack of commitment was the District's decision to stop all further activity in 1987 for a period of three months because of a financial crisis in the District. Due to overspending on the acute budget, the District was unable to rationalize services and release funds promised to mental handicap services. It required the threat of severe financial penalties from the Region to get moving again.

Because of these difficulties, the Mental Handicap Unit lacked a systematic approach to the work that needed to be carried out before the residents could be discharged from the hospital. Many of the staff involved did not seem to anticipate the enormity of the tasks they needed to perform, and this too was a source of delay. Recruitment and induction training for staff took longer and proved to be more difficult, especially as a large number of staff were needed in a short space of time and at the same time when neighbouring districts were also actively recruiting.

The first group home to open in Camberwell was for quite able residents and this glossed over the kinds of issues the District needed to face, leaving them unprepared for the more difficult residents. The failure to select the right staff to get to know residents and then to use that knowledge to create adequate placements explains why, in the end, the District had to make several placements in private psychiatric hospitals.

For their part, regional officers were perhaps too willing to accept at face value the statements from the District that work was going ahead and residents would be transferred on time. As a result, Camberwell still had 11 residents in Darenth Park when it closed, who had to be transferred to the new 'Darenth' ward in Stone House Hospital and to Truscott Villas in August 1988. By the end of September 1988, four residents remained in Dartford and the District anticipated taking them no sooner than March 1989.

Working out new relationships with housing associations

As we saw in Chapter 2, housing subsidies and social security funding could be tapped by involving housing associations in reprovision. Moreover, it was recognized that housing associations had far more experience in building or converting ordinary homes than did the NHS, and it made good sense to use that expertise. Housing associations, too, welcomed this opportunity of working with health authorities. They already had some experience of providing care in the community through their work with local voluntary organizations. The Darenth Park Project allowed them to widen their experience by providing housing for a number of severely handicapped people. Nevertheless, the NHS found difficulty in adjusting to some of the implications.

Officers in the various district mental handicap units tended to see housing associations, naturally enough, as organizations which provided housing – the bricks and mortar of the service. They found the other aspect of housing association work, as the caring landlord, more difficult to accept. Housing associations were concerned with what happened to residents, what kinds of lives they were leading. They saw themselves as having a role to play in the protection of residents' housing rights – residents could not simply be moved from their home at the will of the NHS. NHS officers overlooked the fact that housing association staff now had a responsibility to see that their own housing standards were met. It was no longer the sole responsibility of the NHS to say what was good enough. Housing associations maintained the physical environment of homes as well, and became concerned with what was actually happening to the residents in the community, e.g. the lack of day care arrangements or low staffing levels which made it difficult for residents to get out frequently. Housing associations thus became advocates on behalf of their residents, not just passive house builders.

NHS officers were also initially reluctant to share information about residents, even though some of it had a bearing on the design of houses, e.g. particular behavioural traits might require secure fittings, locks on doors, etc. Over time, these issues were resolved, but at first they did cause friction in the working relationship between the NHS and the housing associations. This was particularly unfortunate in that the NHS did not take advantage of the experience housing associations had in providing community care. Their earlier involvement would have led to a better assessment of the housing needs of residents.

Experience has shown health authorities some of the good sense which lies behind housing association advice. For the associations, the Darenth Park exercise has enabled them to develop much closer relationships with the statutory agencies. They have widened their experience to encompass the design of housing for the severely handicapped, and have learned of the need for a wider variety of housing for people coming out of hospital. Overall, the Darenth Park Project has caught the imagination of housing associations and allowed them to progress much faster than is usual.

A new style of joint management for housing and other services

Two consortia were established in three of the district health authorities; a third agency, already in existence and managing homes for people with a mental handicap, was used to manage the houses in part of one district. A fourth district along with its social services department was setting up a consortium at the time of writing (late 1988). It may well be worth spelling out the nature of these new organizations in some detail.

The Southwark Mental Handicap Consortium was established at the beginning of 1984. It grew out of the approach by Lewisham and North Southwark Health Authority to Cambridge House, a Southwark-based university settlement, to manage a housing scheme the health authority was planning in Southwark. From that meeting came the idea of a conference to consider the creation of a consortium to co-ordinate a borough-wide housing service for the mentally handicapped and to develop and manage the new housing projects. Camberwell Health Authority was then brought into the discussion as were Southwark Social Services. A conference was organized on the theme 'An ordinary life'. From this conference in January 1985 the consortium was established. Initially, it received grants from the Joseph

Rowntree Memorial Trust, the Kings Fund and the Mental Health Foundation. These were used to appoint two development workers, to establish a base at Cambridge House and to begin working with the health authorities and housing associations to develop a housing programme in Southwark.

Legally, the consortium is both a registered charity and a company limited by guarantee. Constitutionally, it is a federative structure composed of two health authorities, Southwark Council, housing associations providing housing in the borough, Southwark Adult Education Institute, Cambridge House, other local organizations and individual members. Its management committee has representatives from each of these so that the consortium is much more than a housing agent for statutory organizations. Not only is it the 'caring landlord', a role carried out on behalf of the housing associations, but it has a wider concern for the well-being of residents and the quality of their lives.

Its membership participates in policy development and in the management of consortium activities through a committee system. Below the management committee are four sub-committees: finance, supported housing, service development and project development. Further, each house has its own project committee as a subordinate group of the supported housing committee.

The consortium has three sources of funds: the charges it makes to residents (the majority of whom claim some form of social security benefit), a hostel deficit grant from the Housing Corporation, and grants from statutory agencies.

The Southwark Consortium has a major stake in co-ordination and joint planning because the Borough contains two health authorities. These, along with the Council's social services department, have in the past tended each to go their own way. The consortium has acted as a neutral meeting point where issues can be discussed between many agencies, so that criticism becomes more acceptable and more constructive. Expertise is shared, especially by the social services department, which has considerable knowledge of running homes. Once the immediate need for housing development was over, consortium members reviewed their objectives and expanded these to consider day care issues and ways in which local people, including those resident in homes, could have a voice in management.

A second consortium was established in Bexley in 1987. It came about largely at the instigation of the district health authority. The local authority, while not objecting, gave very little support. The Bexley Consortium, unlike that in Southwark, was initiated to co-ordinate housing schemes only – there was no intention that it would be concerned with issues beyond housing. The consortium, however, got caught up in wider issues of joint planning between the district health authority and Bexley Council (see Chapter 6), and stated its intention to disband itself in June 1988.

The reasons for this relate largely to the degree of support it received. The consortium was not fully supported by either statutory agency: the local authority did not take up its place on the management committee, and few

NHS officers were convinced of the need for the consortium. The request by the statutory agencies that the consortium take over all management functions of the housing service came much too soon in its existence. The consortium members had considerable doubts as to whether it ought to take over the management of the council's hostels; its objective had been to promote the use of ordinary housing for people with a mental handicap. More importantly, Bexley, unlike Southwark, does not have the wide variety of voluntary organizations and other interested parties, both new and well-established, to support and guide the development of a new organization such as the consortium. The Bexley Consortium was weak in management skills, because it did not have experienced people to draw from its membership.

The third organization, the Providence Project in Lewisham, is quite different from the two consortia. The project began in 1981, when a group of parents and professionals got together to provide accommodation on a different model of care than was then currently available from statutory authorities. At that time, the only type of accommodation available locally was a council hostel. The capital cost of a new home was met largely by the Mayor's appeal which was enough to purchase a home for 12 residents. Several years later, when some of its residents wanted to move to smaller accommodation, the Providence Project was able to get help from a Rotary Club to buy a house. It became apparent that it would be better for them to establish links with housing associations and get financial support from the Housing Corporation.

At the same time, Lewisham and North Southwark Health Authority were looking for an organization to work with them on the housing programme in Lewisham for people coming out of Darenth Park. Officers felt it made more sense to link up with an organization that already had experience of housing management and which had links with local people.

As with the housing associations, NHS officers had to learn that the consortia also wanted a much more direct say in the care of residents. Consortia have strong views on the adequacy of services being offered and the quality of life that results for their clients. One of the values of having a consortium is that through drawing on a variety of local organizations for its membership, it opens up the services offered to its clients to wider community scrutiny.

New management structures

All districts – even those which had some mental handicap services prior to the Darenth Park Project – needed to devise new management structures appropriate to the philosophy of service which emphasized the development of clients' skills and interests and the use of community services. The management systems devised by the districts are very much in a state of development, but some early observations may be made.

The most obvious feature, common to all districts, is the novelty of the kinds of services they are trying to provide. Because of the few group homes that have been provided, the number of experienced staff needed to manage small homes have not been generated. However, this is part of a national problem. In addition, the philosophy of normalization is not simple, even if staff are totally committed to it. The result is that there is some confusion about the roll of staff *vis-à-vis* the residents and what managers should be doing to support staff. In some instances, staff have become discouraged because residents have not shown the improvements anticipated. In others, there seems to be no clear vision of what the objectives of activities are.

Until some of the houses were opened, it was difficult for health authorities to gauge what policies needed to be established for the running of homes and for the protection of both staff and residents. Issues such as handling residents' money – opening accounts, paying rent, handling spending money – become much more complex when the nursing officer and the NHS cashier are not on site, and where the intention is to allow the resident the maximum degree of independence. It can be argued that basic issues like this should have been anticipated and policies established, but that underestimates the amount of transitional work needed simply to get houses opened and clients settled. Other authorities should learn from this experience.

A much greater emphasis should be placed on training, especially in-service training. Most of the districts gave groups of staff a one-week induction course before the houses opened, but this was not made available to those who joined later. In any case, a one-week course is inadequate for the dissemination of knowledge and the acquisition of new skills. The issues which seemed to present the greatest difficulties to staff were how to handle aggressive or violent residents, how to deal safely with drugs, and how to motivate residents.

Because many of the staff do not have a nursing or hospital background, health issues also need special attention, e.g. how to recognize illness in those residents who are often unable to express discomfort or pain? How to lift residents without injuring oneself? How to recognize the side-effects of drugs?

Day care

The absence of day care facilities has been one of the major failings of the project. This includes finding not only places in social education centres but adequate adult education classes or recreation facilities. It is compounded by the seemingly insoluble problem of arranging acceptable transport for people with mobility problems. This has meant that many residents spend considerable amounts of time in their houses, which puts increased pressure on staff to find things for them to do. Developing techniques to help residents to find interesting ways to occupy their time in the house is another area where in-service training could assist staff in their work.

Table 5.1 Staff in Dartford and an inner London district

Age	Dartford	Inner London DHA
Under 20	—	1
20–24	3	34
25–29	8	20
30–34	10	20
35–39	14	12
40–44	24	5
45–49	21	1
50–54	22	—
54–59	16	3
Male staff	20	50
Qualified nurses	51	12

The new staff: home care

In 1983, Darenth Park employed 440 nursing staff to look after 716 residents. By 1988, when the hospital closed, the districts employed more than double that number of staff to look after just over 700 residents.

We attempted to gather information about the new staff being employed in the districts, but in one district alone was there a measurable response rate (≈50%). The basic characteristics of the staff in this district contrast fairly sharply with the staff in Dartford, all of whom were recruited from Darenth Park.

Quite a number of the staff employed in the inner-London district had some relevant work experience: 37 had worked with people with learning disabilities; 22 had previous experience in residential or day care with other client groups; 8 had youth and community work experience; and 12 had other types of voluntary work experience. The staff in Dartford were all recruited from Darenth Park Hospital. In the London districts, 32 staff were recruited through the national press, 50 through the local press and 14 through friends already employed in the service.

A further sharp contrast lies in the length of time staff have been employed by their district. In the London district, only 1 staff member had been employed since 1983, five had been employed in 1986, 16 in 1987 and 73 in 1988 (1 did not reply). This contrasts with Dartford's experience, as shown below:

Before 1970	15
1970–74	31
1975–79	47
1980–84	21
1985–88	6

It is likely that these districts will face quite different problems – one of finding ways of introducing people with fresh ideas into a service that has a high degree of stability, and the other creating continuity in a situation which may have a high turnover of staff.

In brief

We have seen that the new financial incentives and the management changes after 1983 did break the log-jam and in a remarkably short period districts were able to arrange alternative facilities for Darenth Park residents. This was achieved by adopting 'normalization' as a goal and using traditional housing which attracted additional central government financial support. Normalization did, however, bring its own problems. It complicated the range of relationships the NHS had to make with planning and housing departments, with housing associations and consortia. The training problems and need for new management structures were underestimated.

CHAPTER 6

The response of local authorities and local communities

A vain hope

We have already seen that local authorities and local communities responded, at least initially, with a marked lack of enthusiasm to the proposed closure of Darenth Park. The Regional Health Authority had hoped that the closure would be achieved as part of a planned partnership between itself and the local authorities in the catchment area. Local authorities and the NHS were after all under a statutory obligation to collaborate [Section 22(1) of the National Health Service Act 1977]. Joint consultative committees existed at member level. Various circulars instructed authorities how to create joint planning procedures and teams of officers especially to plan for groups like the mentally handicapped [HC(77)17, and HC(83)6].

Academic research on inter-organizational behaviour, however, suggested that such an optimistic view was neither the only or most likely outcome. Challis *et al.* (1988) distinguish what they call an optimistic rational view of the chances of collaboration between public agencies and a pessimistic 'power-dependence/bargaining' perspective. The more optimistic view, adopted by the Region at the outset, was that co-ordination would take place through either authoritative forms of planning such as relying on *Better Services* (DHSS, 1971) norms or through collaborative altruistic activities. The more pessimistic view, presented also by the authors in a previous study of joint planning (Glennerster *et al.*, 1983), suggested that co-ordination is problematic. Most organizations minimize contact and act as protagonists rather than partners: they adjust to each other's activities; bargain and seek mutual advantages from one-off arrangements; and typically buy collaboration or force the other organization to adapt.

The history of the Darenth Park Project is much closer to the second model of inter-organizational activity. Ultimately, the local authorities could not stop the NHS from closing Darenth Park, but they did not have to provide any services that might help the NHS achieve its objective. They could refuse planning permission for new capital developments, though these were open to appeal to central government.

Gradually, central government began to fashion financial incentives that enabled the NHS to buy some kind of cooperation – co-ordination by 'compensation' as Lindblom (1965) calls it. We also observed examples of other categories of 'partisan mutual adjustment', and 'unconditional manipulation' was in evidence. The NHS believed that if residents were placed in a borough the local authority would come under intolerable moral and political pressure to provide services.

As the date of closure advanced, both authorities noted that there were financial gains to be reaped from collaboration as well as political costs to minimize. At this point, we see a growth of 'planned bargaining' (Challis *et al.*, 1988). The growing support for normalization provided a common value basis, whereas in the past divergent organizational interests had been reinforced by professional and philosophical differences about care.

The reluctance of the NHS to admit children to hospital for long-term care meant that there were a growing number of parents with mentally handicapped children in each of the boroughs. They became better organized and groups like Mencap exerted more informed pressure on local councils to provide services for children with a mental handicap. This became extended to facilities for adults.

Nevertheless, other factors were working in the opposite direction. In 1985, four of the seven local authorities in the Darenth Park area found themselves rate-capped. For the first year or so 'creative accounting' sheltered the councils from bringing their expenditure more into line with the government's estimate of what they should be spending. By 1987–8 this was no longer possible. Cuts were now needed and forecasts for the next few years showed that further cuts would be necessary. What modest growth there had been in mental handicap services (in some boroughs, substantial growth) ended, and service provision began to fall.

The new financial policies were not the only central government initiative which upset local government members. Privatization of services and the sale of council houses, to name but two, were seen as attacks on the basic functions of local government and activated considerable and occasionally extremist resistance. Several councils had splits among members as alliances were formed to either resist or bow to government policy. This too directed attention and energy away from the ordinary development of services for particular groups of clients.

Collaboration prior to 1983

The initial stance taken by local authorities in the catchment area was that they were interested in becoming partners in closure of Darenth Park, because they accepted that there were many residents at the hospital who would be suited to care by social services departments. However, for this to happen, health authorities were expected to provide the total necessary capital and revenue upon transfer of responsibilities. The local authorities argued, understandably, that the NHS had been funded to provide for these people in Darenth Park. If they came into the care of another agency funding should follow them. The transfer of responsibility must be accompanied by a transfer of funds.

Regional officers argued that such a transfer was not possible. First, it was not legally possible to transfer funds other than joint finance to local authorities. The NHS could not 'give' money to an agency to provide services for people not needing 'health' care. Secondly, whatever funds were required to be released by the hospital were needed by the NHS itself. The *Care in the Community* circular [HC(83)6], issued in 1983, made possible the transfer of revenue to other agencies to provide services for people coming out of hospital. However, this actually made little difference to the extent of local authority collaboration in this project. In the interim, the health authorities involved in the Darenth Project simply got on with planning, so that when the local authorities did return to the project after 1983, with one exception the districts had more or less completed their plans and were then working on implementing them – finding houses, recruiting staff, and working on relationships with housing associations. There are, however, some examples of joint working between the NHS and local authorities.

Examples of a joint approach

Collaborative planning

Only Greenwich emerged with an agreed comprehensive joint strategy. This came after two years of quarterly meetings, with the Joint Care Working Group (JCWG) chaired by an assistant director of social services. The JCWG succeeded a health care planning team for mental handicap which had been chaired by a health authority member who was also a local councillor. The emergence of the JCWG represented the Council's view that services needed to be planned jointly rather than separately. Both the health authority and the local authority had recently drawn up plans which were fairly different in content and tone. The JCWG was to reconcile these two documents to ensure that service developments would be complementary.

The two statutory authorities had a quite different view about the size and type of provision based on divergent philosophies of care. The DHA used the *Better Services* (DHSS, 1971) norms (55 beds per 100 000) and added to them known shortfalls in local authority provision and additional provision for short-term care. The local authority, however, thought the DHA's views excessive. A second discrepancy existed regarding the local authority's wish to make part of its provision suitable for severely handicapped people, whereas the NHS considered that the local authority should be concerned solely with the more able.

The District accepted that the facilities for which plans existed would still not be adequate for those residents of Darenth Park for whom it was responsible. They therefore began contacting local estate agents to try to find suitable properties. This interested the social services department considerably, as this represented a very different model of care from existing or planned NHS provision, and one which it saw as coming within its range of responsibility. There was a 'boundary problem', however. By the end of 1985, some degree of compromise had been reached which recognized that the health authority should retain responsibility for the more severely handicapped coming out of hospital, and possibly for those still in the community. This was the basis of the *quid pro quo*. The health authority was willing to accept this if they were to begin planning again.

This truce was brought into question when, at the end of April 1986, plans for the development of the 48-place residential centre and a 90-place day centre at the Royal Herbert site had to be scrapped, because the Region had received what was termed a 'generous' offer by a supermarket chain (not Sainsburys) for the site. The District's health care planning team was reconvened to inform the local authority and voluntary organizations of this and to present to them alternative proposals.

The local authority did not react well to this. To some extent officers felt that they had been made fools of by the health authority. They had loyally supported the Royal Herbert development in public consultation and through the local authority planning process, not because they liked it – it violated almost all of their philosophy of care – but because the DHA seemed determined to go ahead. All this now seemed in vain.

The health care planning team meeting took no decision, but allowed a few weeks for comments on these new proposals. One month later the Joint Care Working Group met. This meeting was attended by the Director of Greenwich Social Services, and he and his colleagues protested that they were being presented with a *fait accompli* by the DHA yet again. They saw the need to change plans, making possible a radical rethink of the overall service position in the Borough. The Borough's complaints were that:

● negotiations about the new site had been going on for at least 4–5 months, but the local authority had not been involved or even informed;
● recent DHSS guidance emphasized the importance of joint planning of local services. The action of both the DHA and the Region made nonsense of such guidance.

The social services department objected to the proposed concentration of 32 people on one site, especially as they would be the most handicapped residents. Social services officers put in a bid to manage the additional places now to be provided in ordinary housing, claiming that they had the experience and established management procedures to support group homes. To further these schemes, it suggested a joint resettlement team of one local authority and one health service officer to produce plans and to turn these into services. More dramatically, the director of social services put forward the case of the social services department himself. The District was marginally sympathetic, but it was intensely aware that the closure of Darenth Park was only 22 months away, and that the likelihood of providing enough accommodation was not very good. However, rather than reject the Borough's views out of hand, the NHS officers agreed to consult the Region to see if there was enough time to rethink their services.

By July, the proposed plans put forward to the April health care planning team and May JCWG meetings had been modified, and now consisted of 20 places at the British Hospital for Mothers and Babies site and 12 places in two purpose-built bungalows at the Goldie Leigh site, thus lessening the concentration of residents. The District hoped that the remainder of the Goldie Leigh site would be sold for ordinary housing, thereby integrating the bungalows into a local community. The day centre was to be reduced to accommodate 45 with the proviso that the Region provided capital for a further 45 places if it were needed. Two resettlement officers, one from each statutory agency, were appointed to implement these plans. At the end of 1986, the JCWG officially became the permanent Joint Planning Group on Mental Handicap Services, and by mid-1987 had agreed a joint statement of strategy for the next four years of service development.

The withdrawal from the Royal Herbert site had provided an opportunity to rethink service philosophy. Other factors were also at work:

- The consultant psychiatrist retired in the middle of 1985. This meant one less voice to speak up for a more traditional, medically oriented service.
- A new UGM for Priority Care Services was appointed in May 1986, whose remit included mental handicap services. He had worked in an area where health and social services had collaborated together to develop new mental handicap services based on ordinary housing. He was sympathetic to the social services model of care and to their claim for expertise in managing that type of service.
- A new full-time psychologist was appointed to the mental handicap service. She created a committee to assess the Greenwich residents in Darenth Park which showed that they were younger and had a much wider range of abilities than had previously been thought.
- The District had received funds from the DHSS to develop a new facility for children – under DA(83)3, *Getting Mentally Handicapped Children out of Hospital* (DHSS, 1983c). This unit was run with operational policies close to the principles of normalization, with care plans for each resident, and this gave confidence to the District about providing services based on a different model of care

This coincidence of events, which occurred roughly within 6–12 months, led to the only instance where a significant number of Darenth Park residents were transferred across to the care of a social services department (along with the associated costs of revenue and capital).

Collaboration through privatization

Bexley provides another model of collaboration – privatization. At the time of writing, consultations were taking place on a proposal to provide a joint residential service by a private organization. This was the culmination of attempts over six years to find ways for the two statutory agencies to cooperate. The health authority had relied totally on Darenth Park for adults and Goldie Leigh for children. There were no local health services for people with a mental handicap and no local tradition of member support for such services. The local authority had some, though largely for people with moderate disabilities. Day care services were provided for the more handicapped, but these were limited and still excluded some adults on the grounds that they were too difficult to manage.

When Bexley became a district health authority in 1982, a Joint Care Planning Group (JCPG) for mental handicap services was among the first of such groups to be established. The District needed to make headway in developing services for the Darenth Park residents, but it wanted to do this in the wider context of comprehensive community mental handicap services. The JCPG began meeting in early 1983. Within a year the DHA had produced a draft comprehensive strategy for all mental handicap services, but the local authority was not able either to respond to it or to produce a draft plan for its own services. The JCPG seemed to be drifting along without accomplishing anything, and it was eventually dissolved by the new district general manager (DGM) at the end of 1985. In its place, he established a task force, much smaller in membership and whose focus was solely on progressing plans for the Darenth Park residents. Joint working discussions now took place in the Joint Consultative Committee which soon issued a statement of intent to create a joint service and a joint strategy. This engendered no action but was a marker at member level that some arrangement needed to be worked out.

Both statutory authorities were experiencing changes in personnel at senior levels. Bexley Health Authority had created a joint structure for mental handicap and community health services in 1982, but appointments to new posts were only made gradually: a project officer was appointed in 1984 to develop and implement plans for the Darenth Park residents; a unit administrator, covering both mental handicap and community services, was appointed around the same time; a unit general manager for mental handicap and mental health was appointed in mid-1986; and a divisional manager for mental handicap services was appointed, though not until January 1988. The consequence of this slow build up to the management structure was that decisions about the nature of the service were made fairly low down in the organization and not all of the wider implications were seen. Furthermore, in early 1987, the DGM was dismissed and another appointed, as well as a new director of finance and, in 1988, a new director of planning.

Within the local authority, there were also a number of personnel changes. An assistant chief social services officer, responsible for research and development, was appointed in mid-1986. Over a period of time, vacancies occurred in the posts of two most senior social services officers and the Director of Housing and Personnel Services. These vacancies brought into play senior staff from the Chief Executive and the finance director, whose central concerns were to get the issues resolved at minimum cost. Only one of these officers was concerned with debates about the nature of care. The assistant chief social services officer, within months of his arrival, produced a paper suggesting how local authority services could be developed at no additional cost to the Council, through the involvement of an independent organization to provide services on a contractual basis. This would allow clients to claim a higher level of social security benefits. With these savings, the Council could expand the Community Mental Handicap Team (CMHT), provide a better management structure for its own service – which would put greater emphasis on developing the potential of clients – and increase day care.

These proposals recognized several important factors. First, local authority services needed to be both improved and expanded. The CMHT register was showing an increased demand for both residential and day care from children completing education and being transferred to adult services, and from ageing parents who were increasingly concerned about their declining ability to look after their sons or daughters. The Council had relied completely on Darenth Park for adult short-term care. Since 1984, when this was no longer available, the Council had done very little to develop an in-borough service for respite short-term or emergency care. Mencap was effectively reminding councillors of the needs of people with a mental handicap, and their families.

Secondly, by showing how such developments could be undertaken without requiring additional Council funds, the officers offered an inducement to members to agree to an expansion of services, something members would not be willing to fund without tapping external resources. The involvement of an outside organization was another inducement. The Council could be seen to respond to central government's philosophy that local authorities should oversee rather than directly provide services (the Secretary of State's speech at Buxton to Directors of Social Services, 1984).

Thirdly, by proposing that residential services be provided by an outside agency, their aim was to overcome the concern felt by local authority officers and members about the health authority's approach. In their view, the DHA could not afford to maintain the kinds of mental handicap services it currently envisaged because of the costs incurred by high staffing levels. The DHA's service was based on a significant contribution towards costs by the clients claiming social security benefits. Local authority officers thought that the Bexley Mental Handicap Consortium, set up largely by the health authority to manage services in a way which would allow the clients' benefits to be maximized, was simply too close to the health authority to be independent. The local authority feared that at some stage, local DHSS officers would decide the consortium was only a front for receiving benefits, and therefore cut them off. At that point, the DHA would not be able to meet the full costs of the service and the local authority would somehow have to pick up the pieces.

The paper produced by the assistant chief social services officer eventually appeared as a brief proposal for a joint service in February 1987. The first problem the local authority faced was to convince the DHA that the services then being implemented were going to be too expensive. This was a matter of some dispute. The District's financial plans assumed that the cost of services would fall over a five-year period to a level not above that of the dowry, and that staffing levels would be curtailed as residents adapted to living outside the hospital and became able to do more for themselves. However, the local authority did not believe this. A new director of finance was appointed to the DHA after a financial crisis and he was in agreement with the local authority that the District's mental handicap services were too expensive. He in turn was able to convince the District's other senior managers that changes had to be made and an agreement on a joint service with the local authority would represent the best way forward.

A brief strategy proposal for a joint approach, with services provided by an outside agency, was put to the Housing and Social Services Committee of the local authority and the DHA during the summer of 1987 and was approved by both as the basis for further detailed negotiations. To show the level of political importance attached to this issue, the leader of Bexley Council attended the DHA meeting to speak in support of the proposal. A Joint Officer Working Party (JOWP) was set up, but initially most of the work was done in two sub-groups, one concerned with care policies and the other with organization and management. The Community Health Council (CHC), Bexley Mencap and the regional health authority were invited to become observers to the JOWP. The CHC was informed by Bexley Health Authority that it would not be formally consulted because the authority did not consider that a change of service was involved. The Region intervened and suggested consultations, and it was agreed that the CHC would be involved in the plans to implement the policy.

Separate from those two working groups, the local authority pursued its intention to engage a voluntary organization to take over management responsibility for residential services. Three national organizations were approached and expressed interest. No final agreement was reached because of difficulties over issues relating to staff. The local authority had decided that total protection would be given to its existing staff, and no voluntary organization was willing to have its staffing policies decided for it. In addition, the local authority wanted to move quickly, which proved impossible.

At the same time, the DHA pushed the virtues of the existing consortium. The consortium had already been established, employed housing staff and had taken on the housing management responsibilities in a satisfactory way. Moreover, the local DHSS had agreed residents were eligible for the higher levels of board and lodgings allowances granted to clients in registered care homes, thereby proving local authority fears that the consortium would be seen as a front for the health authority to be groundless. On this basis, the local authority agreed, towards the end of 1987, that the consortium could act as the third party. Negotiations were then opened with the consortium, and senior officers from the local authority and the health authority attended a consortium meeting in November 1987 to discuss some of the issues involved.

Then both the DHA and the local authority made what is now recognized as two mistakes. They assumed that the consortium was a creation of the health authority, and therefore would do exactly what the health authority officers asked it to do. Negotiations with the consortium were expected to be fairly straightforward and it was hoped that an interim agreement could be reached by January 1988. In reality, there were major differences between the consortium and the statutory authorities. The consortium had been set up to develop and manage ordinary houses, and it was now being asked to take on the Council's three hostels. So far, it had worked with housing associations and the health authority, and it was now being asked to work with the local authority, bringing in a new set of working relationships. The consortium had also intended working towards the gradual introduction of its own care staff, but it was now being asked to employ or be responsible through secondment for all local authority and DHA staff working in mental handicap residential services. Speed was all important.

The consortium itself had weaknesses. First, its management committee was lacking in expertise, especially in the management of independent organizations. This reflected the lack of voluntary activity in Bexley, its most active members being health service officers (or ex-health service officers) and housing association representatives. Secondly, its members were volunteers, who gave up their evenings for meetings, no match for officers deeply immersed in the politics of the situation. Thirdly, it was a very young organization that was asked to take on major negotiations with statutory agencies.

Many of the members of the committee had been closely involved with the development of the District's new services and were understandably reluctant to see them change in a way which they considered would lower their quality. The consortium was being asked to take on responsibility for a model of service totally different from what it was used to. Members of the consortium's management committee were well aware of the earlier negotiations with national voluntary organizations over work which the consortium was already doing. They felt that they had been treated fairly shabbily and that the early discussions on a jointly managed residential service had been carried out in an underhanded way.

By Christmas 1987, the local authority and the health authority had agreed on a model of care which in principle was closer to that of the consortium.

The key issue then became the management structure. The consortium submitted a management structure which, from the viewpoint of the JOWP, was too extensive and therefore too expensive. The local authority (and possibly DHA) used this to show its lack of faith in the consortium to manage effectively the services they were asking it to take on, a much more general criticism than one limited to the management structure. Negotiations which had been going on during the first four months of 1988 were broken off by the

JOWP in May 1988. Two senior officers attended a consortium management committee meeting at which they announced that the health and local authorities had reached agreement with a private non-profit organization to take on management responsibilities, and hence, in June 1988, the consortium began proceedings to dissolve itself. At the time of writing (early 1989) this was being reconsidered.

The organization with which the statutory authorities had reached agreement was a private company limited by guarantee, owned by the former director of housing and personal services of Bexley Council. Social Policy Management Services (SPMS) Ltd would obviously be more to the liking of the local authority than the consortium, as it was established specifically for the purpose of taking on residential services within the framework desired by the JOWP. Meanwhile, the DHA had agreed in March to become involved in the consultation process on the basis of the consortium being the voluntary organization mentioned in the proposed change of service, although it argued that consultation was about the principle not the organization.

As part of this consultation process, the CHC held a public meeting in July on whether the two statutory services should combine to provide a single residential service. The meeting was attended by a number of people with a mental handicap, and parents and care staff. It was a difficult meeting, as it was concerned with consultation on a health authority document, yet most of the issues related to local authority responsibilities and intentions, such as the inadequacy of day care and of special needs day care, the role hostels would play in the new service, the basis on which clients would be moved from hostel to an ordinary house or the reverse, and the length of time needed to generate a pool of resources for service development. It was a less than harmonious meeting, indicating some of the hostility generated by recent events in the Borough and disagreement with the concept of privatizing residential services.

This meeting allowed the CHC to assess the public mood as regards the proposed service change. It conveyed its views to the district health authority which then produced an assessment of all comments received by the close of the consultation period in July. In that document the health authority attempted to offer reassurance to the CHC and others that the main points of disagreement were being discussed and resolved. These issues related to the question of the security of tenure of residents in houses managed by SPMS, the nature of SPMS as an organization, an alternative proposal by a group of parents for a different organization, the philosophy of care which the new agency would follow, the establishment of a consumer council to help monitor services provided, and several other issues. Because of the CHC's objections to the initial proposals, the regional health authority became involved as a participant in further negotiations. The local authority and health authority produced a joint service specification and draft code of practice which spelt out how the service would operate. A further CHC meeting was held in October 1988 and, at that time, although the CHC still opposed the proposals, CHC members were pleased with the major advances made regarding the framework for a new service. A number of points were still outstanding and, because the proposal to contract-out services to a privately owned organization was so recent, the CHC was reluctant to give formal approval until all points had been clarified and all documents finalized. These views were conveyed to the November DHA meeting.

The local authority signed a contract with SPMS in September 1988 and in April 1989 the health authority did so as well.

Bromley

In a third borough, Bromley, negotiations were at the time of writing being conducted to create a single statutory service. Bromley was chosen by the Audit Commission for a trial audit based on the ideas found in its report on community care. Several changes have made the negotiations more likely to succeed. Over the past 10 years, the local authority, which could no longer gain admission for its residents to the hospital, learned how to cope with more handicapped people. Differences in philosophy of care have lessened, with both statutory agencies seeing that at least a part of their services could be provided in ordinary housing. Now that Bromley Health Authority has transferred all of its residents from Darenth Park, both agencies have a much clearer picture of what their existing commitments are. The social services department and the DHA developed a joint children's service. Three houses have joint staff appointments and three have mainly NHS staff because of the degree of physical handicap of the children. The closure of an old children's hospital and an underused children's home provided the opportunity for this. The DHA is also responsible for the closure of a nearby mental illness hospital and this has increased the scope for negotiation with the local authority.

Service developments in the community

Involvement with the Darenth Park Project was only part of local authorities' concerns about the development of services for people with learning disabilities. Several local authorities were already actively increasing services for their client groups when the Darenth Park Project began in 1978. Over the 10 years of the project, local authorities continued to develop their own services for people who had never been in hospital. Closure acted as a catalyst, though the pace of change of some authorities slowed down as constraints on local government finance began to bite. Table 6.1 lists the changes which have taken place in local authority services. The range of types of scheme is impressive.

Table 6.1 Local authority developments in detail

	1978	1984	1988	Better Services norms, 1988 LA population estimate
Dartford and Gravesham	not available	25 hostels	24 hostels	
		9 group homes	9 group homes	
		10 vol. in-borough	18 vol. in-borough	
		35 P/V	36 P/V	
			1 assisted landlady	
		140 day care	162 day care	
		20 special care	34 special care	
Totals		79 residential	88 residential	168 residential
		160 day care	196 day care	160 day care
Bromley	25 hostel	46 hostels	24 hostels	
	35 agency	4 group homes	29 group homes	
	225 day care	28 vol. in-borough	55 out-of-borough P/V	
		3 shared care	8 family placements	
		41 vol. outside	48 vol. in-borough	
		3 in other LA facilities	10 private in-borough	
		19 private	11 live-in carers	
		240 day care	276 day care	
		40 special care	40 special care	
Totals	60 residential	144 residential	181 residential	224 residential
	225 day care	280 day care	316 day care	387 day care

Bexley

38 hostels 25 P/V 163 day care	38 hostels 4 semi-independent units 25 P/V 202 day care 18 special care	42 hostels 4 semi-independent living 9 group homes 5 independent tenancies 60 out-of-borough P/V 232 day care 18 special care	164 residential 285 day care
Totals 63 residential 163 day care	67 residential 220 day care	120 residential 250 day care	

Greenwich

42 hostels 16 sheltered housing 49 P/V 235 day care 30 special care	42 hostels 21 sheltered housing 7 group homes 64 P/V 3 boarding out 2 CSV-supported independent living 220 day care 45 special care	42 hostels 22 sheltered housing 3 group homes 56 P/V out-of-borough 40–45 boarding out/family placements 5 CSV-supported independent living 6 shared tenancies supported by 2 group homes Project Teams 273 day care 45 special care	161 residential 280 day care
Totals 107 residential 265 day care	139 residential 265 day care	174–9 residential 318 day care	

continued

Table 6.1 continued

	1978	1984	1988	Better Services norms, 1988 LA population estimate
Lewisham				
	30 hostels	68 hostels	68 hostels	
	4 group homes	8 group homes	14 group homes	
			14 flatlets	
		30 boarding out	28 boarding out	
	80 P/V	17 vol. in-borough	33 P/V in-borough	
		78 P/V out-of-borough	64 P/V out-of-borough	
	160 day care	260 day care	280 day care	
	20 special care	20 special care		
Totals	114 residential	201 residential	221 residential	173 residential
	180 day care	280 day care	280 day care	299 day care
Lambeth				
	20 hostels	12 hostels	17 hostels	
		8 group homes	18 group homes	
	10 P/V in-borough	40 vol. in-borough	77 P/V in-borough	
	60 P/V out-of-borough	90 P/V out-of-borough	104 P/V out-of-borough (including some children)	
		12 sheltered housing	12 sheltered housing	
		6 boarding out		
	150 day care	150 day care	150 day care	
	15 special needs	33 special needs	53 special needs	
Totals	90 residential	168 residential	228 residential	182 residential
	165 day care	183 day care	203 day care	316 day care

Southwark

36 hostels	48 hostels	80 hostels	
4 group homes	4 group homes	12 group homes	
50–60 P/V	53 P/V	18 P/V in-borough	
		1 other LA	
		2 boarding out	
		68 P/V out-of-borough	
180 day care	180 day care	232 day care attendance	
14 special care	14 special care	9 day care out-of-borough	
Totals 90–100 residential	105 residential	181 residential	158 residential
194 day care	194 day care	241 day care	273 day care

1 *Core and cluster.* This is the development of several units which are geographically close (not necessarily next to each other), the core unit having more specialized staff, and the other nearby units functioning independently but drawing on the core unit for additional help if needed. Originally, these schemes used older community housing.
2 *Small group homes.* The use of community housing for 2–4 people living together, with either 24-hour staff, day staff, peripatetic staff or no staff. The residents are encouraged to run the house and perform as many tasks as they are able to.
3 *Home care.* This scheme provides relief to families caring for a member who is doubly incontinent or has disturbed behaviour. The development officer recruits and trains workers who link in with a family, get to know all of its members and learn how to handle the member with a handicap. The family may book relief care up to two and in some cases three weeks per annum. The family contribution to the cost of this service is £1 per half day up to £21 per week.
4 *Semi-independent living.* The provision of small group homes or individual living arrangements near a hostel or staffed group home, so that residents may easily call for help if needed.
5 *Hostels.* A much larger group of people living together (up to 30), usually with 24-hour staff coverage.
6 *Family care/boarding out/adult care.* These schemes cover individual placements in a family setting or in a small lodging house. When part of a family setting, the home owners are expected to provide care and support as well as board and lodgings. The DHSS makes some payments for this type of service, and local authorities may often top this up depending on the level of care being provided.

In brief

Overall, local authorities and the NHS began the Darenth Park venture as protagonists rather than collaborators. Many of the interactions academic theorists predicted are observable. Monetary incentives by the NHS came too late to facilitate the movement of residents from NHS to local authority care. Financial disincentives caused by general central government funding were making day care and other provisions increasingly difficult. This is a major weakness. Nevertheless, some mutually beneficial schemes began to be realized. One of the interesting features of the later period was the emergence of joint management arrangements, sometimes through a completely separate agency. This seemed to remove some of the barriers that existed to direct collaboration between statutory authorities. In the end, it has been more influential than joint finance itself.

CHAPTER 7

Getting people ready for the service

The residents

So far, we have been concerned with the bureaucratic politics that were the central feature of the closure. What of the people one might have thought would be the central focus – the residents? They have been the subject of detailed research by Lorna Wing and her colleagues at the MRC Social Psychiatry Research Unit at the Institute of Psychiatry in London. That research team began their work in 1980 when there were nearly 900 residents. They have kindly made available breakdowns of the social and behavioural characteristics of the residents whom they have been following since that date. Their research is reported in detail elsewhere (Wing, 1989).

Of the 888 people participating in the study, Wing records that 507 were men and 381 were women. Of these, 172 were in their 60s, 112 were in their 70s and 35 were over 80 years old – one was over 90 (see Table 7.1). About 60% of all residents originated from within the hospital's catchment area. About half the residents had lived in the hospital for over 25 years. A total of 14% of the residents (122 people) were unable to walk independently. About 40% (350 people) had some form of impaired social interaction. About half had no contact with friends or relations outside the hospital, especially the older people; but the younger residents had more visits. Nearly two-fifths of all the residents needed help with feeding, washing and dressing. About a quarter suffered from severe incontinence. A quarter could not indicate even simple needs. Altogether, about one-third were categorized by Wing as having severe behaviour problems. The younger residents had more severe handicaps – reflecting the changing admissions criteria of our time. Many older residents would not have been admitted to institutional care more recently. Thus those who were least handicapped had lived longest in the institution and the youngest were most in need of intensive care. The presence of severe behaviour problems was recorded for more than two-thirds of those aged 30 or under.

The fact that about 44% of residents did *not* suffer from major disabling conditions or behaviour problems meant that in the early stages of the project

Table 7.1 The age and sex of residents in 1980 (in percentages)[a]

	Lambeth/ Southwark	Lewisham	Greenwich/ Bexley	Dartford/ Gravesham	Bromley	All districts
Age group						
0–19	2.2	3.8	1.1	16.7	—	3.8
20–29	14.7	24.1	17.2	15.1	13.8	16.8
30–39	12.5	14.3	14.2	20.6	11.6	14.3
40–49	10.7	6.0	11.6	13.5	13.8	11.2
50–59	18.8	21.8	15.0	15.1	21.0	17.9
60–69	18.8	21.0	22.1	11.9	20.3	19.3
70–79	16.1	6.8	13.5	6.3	16.6	12.6
80+	6.2	2.2	5.3	0.8	2.9	4.1
Sex						
Male	61.6	45.9	50.7	57.9	57.1	57.1
Female	38.4	32.2	49.3	42.1	42.9	42.9
Total number of residents	224	133	267	138	126	888

[a] For whom full details were available.

the hospital community benefited from a good deal of social interaction. There were longstanding friendships and a fairly permissive attitude to relationships. The wards (see Chapter 3) had been 'sectorized', to contain all those who originally came from the same borough. This had split old friendships but new ones were established. The more able residents had some degree of independence and personal space. The more disabled were the subject of much more attention, but their standards of living were low. The wards contained very different age groups. Residents from Lewisham, Greenwich and Bexley had been there longest. The residents in the new sectorized wards included many 'non-catchment' residents to whom no original address was attached. The residents in the various boroughs/wards also differed considerably in the severity of their handicaps (see Tables 7.2–7.4).

Table 7.2 Residents and their type of disability by borough, 1980

	Lambeth/ Southwark	Greenwich/ Lewisham	Bexley	Dartford/ Gravesham	Bromley	All
Wheelchair-bound	25	15	40	30	12	122
Totally or almost totally blind	9	16	7	10	2	44
Blind	1	1	1	0	0	3
Blind and deaf	2	1	2	1	0	6

Table 7.3 The behaviour patterns of residents in 1980

Type of behaviour	Lambeth/ Southwark	Lewisham	Greenwich/ Bexley	Dartford/ Gravesham	Bromley	Total
Socially impaired with behaviour problems	40 (17.4%)	37 (27.8%)	56 (21.0%)	28 (22.2%)	25 (18.1%)	186 (20.9%)
Socially impaired with no behaviour problems	40 (17.9%)	23 (17.3%)	41 (15.3%)	37 (29.4%)	23 (16.7%)	164 (18.4%)
Sociable with behaviour problems	43 (19.2%)	15 (11.3%)	44 (16.5%)	14 (11.1%)	31 (22.5%)	147 (16.6%)
Sociable with no behaviour problems	101 (45.0%)	58 (43.5%)	126 (47.2%)	47 (37.3%)	59 (42.7%)	391 (44.0%)

Table 7.4 Residents' length of stay in hospital in 1980

Years	Lambeth/ Southwark	Lewisham	Greenwich/ Bexley	Dartford/ Gravesham	Bromley	Total
0–1	2	0	0	6	0	8
1–5	15	6	14	16	15	66
6–10	12	12	16	18	5	63
11–15	11	12	33	13	4	73
16–20	39	21	43	28	17	148
21–25	23	15	27	20	13	98
26–30	8	8	9	7	7	39
31–35	9	6	16	3	5	39
36–40	14	4	11	3	11	43
41–45	15	11	18	4	13	61
46–50	47	24	48	2	33	154
51–55	8	6	13	2	7	36
56–60	11	6	8	2	4	31
61–65	8	2	6	1	3	20
66–70	1	0	1	1	0	3
71–75	0	0	1	0	1	2
76–80	1	0	3	0	0	4
Total	224	133	267	126	138	888

Preparation for the move

Bureaucratic changes

Two kinds of organizational preparation were made in the long process of moving residents. The first was the sectorization of the wards, as we have already described and which is discussed further in Chapter 8. The next steps were:

- Getting agreement with the districts about how many residents each should take.

- Assigning residents to districts which kept changing their boundaries through the project and were not the same as borough boundaries.
- Assessing the residents and forming groups of those who would live together.
- Finding placements for those residents who had particular requests or whose needs were too special for their assigned district to provide.

We consider these practical bureaucratic issues in turn.

Getting agreement on numbers

Regional officers intended to use the closure of Darenth Park to reduce the traditional dependence on the hospital by local authorities for admissions based on social criteria. Although in some local authorities local provision for mentally handicapped people had improved, the hospital still had a large proportion of residents who could fairly easily live in alternative provision in their local communities – they had no medical or nursing reason to be in hospital. According to *Better Services* (DHSS, 1971) norms, the seven districts using Darenth Park 'should' have provided 825 beds instead of the 988 places then available in the hospital. The decision was taken to fund no more than 825 places in the seven districts. This seemed reasonable because of the age structure of the hospital's residents. Statistical analysis showed that about 30 deaths would occur annually over the next 5–8 years, and that this would result in a decline in the number of residents needing to be accommodated – more or less matching the number of places the Region would fund.

The non-catchment residents posed another problem. Agreement had already been reached among the districts that the non-catchment residents would be distributed in proportion to the resident population of the districts. However, it had been shown (see Chapter 5; Korman and Glennerster, 1985) that the formula, when taken in conjunction with the number of catchment residents each district had, would result in some districts having places but no residents and others too many residents for the number of places they would be providing. Negotiations between regional officers and districts resulted in this problem being resolved by both Bromley and Lewisham and North Southwark taking more non-catchment residents than they would according to the formula, and Bexley being allowed to take non-catchment residents because of the difficulty the district was having in finding suitable sites.

Attaching residents to districts

Once the numbers had been agreed, it was then left to those districts taking non-catchment residents to choose which ones they would take. By the end of 1986, of those not yet assigned to a district, 16 were thought to have severe behaviour problems. Five of these residents were subject to detention orders under the Mental Health Act. This problem was brought to the attention of the Steering Group in October 1986. It was thought unlikely that the districts would willingly take responsibility for these residents, because they would

Table 7.5 Mismatch of residents and places

Sector	Catchment residents	Agreed number of noncatchment	Total number	Number of places being provided
Dartford/Gravesham	80	40	120	120
Bromley	36	50	86	144
Greenwich/Bexley	137	72	209	214
Lewisham	39	31	70	24
Lambeth/Southwark	150	91	214	120[a]

[a] These places were for Camberwell/West Lambeth residents, including those sector residents who belonged to the N. Southwark part of Lewisham and North Southwark.

probably require high staffing levels, they had no links to districts, and the districts themselves were becoming concerned about the overall costs of reprovision. In light of these factors, a special meeting was called. In preparation for it, a consultant psychiatrist and the leader of the special development team assessed the 16 residents, so that information about them could be given to district representatives. These were based on medical records, not personal assessments of the individuals involved.

The meeting at which these allocations to districts took place could scarcely be described as congenial. District representatives recognized that the hospital could not close until these residents had alternative places. But assigning these residents to districts could not have come at a more difficult time for the districts. Only one district, Dartford and Gravesham, planned to cater for residents with special needs within its main development, Archery House. The remaining districts would have to make special arrangements, which in several cases meant acquiring additional houses. Some of these residents would also require more personal and closer supervision which inevitably meant higher costs. Furthermore, there was a time factor involved – the hospital was due to close within 15 months and the districts had doubts of whether they could organize special services in time, particularly when they were already under pressure to maintain the existing programme of discharges.

Regional officers, however, were adamant that the meeting would resolve the issue of district responsibility for these residents. Districts were reminded that they had been required to make provision for the whole range of mental handicap services (not a particularly good argument, since districts only intended to plan services for those residents they knew they would be taking). The possibility of extra funds for catering for these residents was held out to the districts, and they agreed a distribution. Even so, uncertainty remained. How much extra money would there be? The Region had only stated that there was a possibility of extra funds. Were these residents now to count as part of the districts' agreed number of residents or were they extra? This latter point was of some importance, for if they counted as part of a district's agreed number, that district would not replace residents who died in hospital with others from the non-allocated list. As this turned out, the majority of the 16 residents involved simply fitted into existing planned district services – group homes, hostels or residential centres requiring no special facilities. Two of these received treatment and assessment in the Mental Impairment Evaluation and Treatment Service unit before going to their districts. One resident became the subject of a special development team project. Two others are temporary residents of Archery House, waiting for services to be designed and provided for them in their home district. One went to a private placement out of district to be near his family. Therefore, despite being labelled as having special needs, many moved into ordinary facilities.

Assessing residents

It was left to each district to decide how to assess their residents. Each district was more or less seeking the same information – mobility, self-care skills, interests and hobbies, recreational skills, ability to handle money, awareness of danger, ability to communicate, friendships – but tended to go about getting this information in different ways.

Residents of Darenth Park had already been assessed twice. The first was by the social work assessment team, appointed through joint finance in 1980, and completed by a social worker from Bromley who remained at the hospital after other team members had left. This assessment was concerned principally with the appropriate kinds of residential accommodation needed, but it was not used by many districts because the range of residential options proposed did not match the types of facilities being planned by districts. In particular, many more residents were to live in group homes and almost none would be going to a 'hospital'. Some district staff also saw this assessment as failing to show any potential for development among the residents; this may or may not be true, but it was how it was viewed.

The second assessment was carried out by Dr Lorna Wing and her team as part of the funded research on Darenth Park clients (as is mentioned below, these assessments were used by two districts). In general, however, the districts wanted to assess their residents themselves. Assessment was a way of getting to know the residents as people, and respecting their individuality. As so many of the district staff were new, it is also questionable whether they were actually aware of these previous assessments.

Dartford and Gravesham had perhaps the easiest task, since their senior staff were appointed from Darenth Park and already knew their residents quite well. None the less, they undertook multidisciplinary reviews of each resident involving medical, nursing and training department staff.

Bromley developed a 'Moving-on Committee' which had responsibility for assessing and grouping the residents prior to discharge. Shortly after the 1982 restructuring, Bromley had appointed a core of senior staff to plan their services: a director of nursing services (as the district already had a children's unit and a hostel for mildly handicapped women), a clinical psychologist, and a head of client training. These officers, along with the senior nursing officer for the Bromley sector and the Bromley social worker (both working at Darenth Park), and a representative from the training department at the hospital, formed the Moving-on Committee. The committee reviewed each resident, inviting the ward sister/charge nurse who knew the resident best to participate in the review. A form was devised covering the main areas of the resident's abilities and life which would be helpful in placing the resident in suitable accommodation. From 1983 onward, staff appointed to the client training department and to the psychology service worked part of the time at Darenth Park, getting to know the residents of the sector. They too contributed to the reviews of the residents. Bromley's consultant psychiatrist was also involved, giving psychiatric reviews as necessary. Reviews were reassessed closer to the time residents moved out to monitor any changes which had taken place. In this way, the Moving-on Committee was able to get an overall view of their residents and reach decisions about the most appropriate placements for them. This overview of the residents contributed to the development of the District's philosophy of care, which was significantly modified during 1984 to allow a larger variety of living situations for those residents capable of independent living and to 'deinstitutionalize' the District's 72-place residential centre.

This innovation proved important for others. A Moving-on Committee was also set up in Greenwich, largely at the instigation of the clinical psychologist who was appointed in 1985. Wing's disablement assessment schedule (DAS) of the residents was used as a foundation from which further ratings assessments could be made. An interview schedule was designed which incorporated the results of the DAS assessment. This schedule asked questions about mobility, continence, self-help skills, communication skills, educational ability, behaviour, medical information, length of stay in hospital, and whether the resident was under a restrictive order. A further set of questions dealt with the resident's social network, friends in and out of Darenth Park, family contacts, sociability, day care and leisure activities, work experience, use of community facilities, and potential for development of home-making skills. The interviewer was also asked to make some notes of his/her personal impression of the resident so that they would be able to recall the particular resident at future meetings. These questionnaires were used in interviews with both Darenth Park ward staff and the resident where possible.

In Greenwich the Moving-on Committee consisted of the clinical psychologist, a psychology technician, two social workers – one of whom worked at Goldie Leigh – two community nurses and a welfare visitor from Greenwich Mencap. The senior nursing officer for the Greenwich/Bexley sector at Darenth Park also attended when needed as did the Darenth Park social worker and other nursing and training staff. Each member of the committee undertook interviews with six to eight residents.

Other districts used their community mental handicap teams (CMHTs) to assess the Darenth Park residents – Bexley, Lewisham and North Southwark, and Camberwell. These were the only staff who were available and knowledgeable enough to carry out the assessments. In Lewisham and North Southwark, some service needs assessments had already been carried out in 1981–2 by the central staff planning the new services, but these had been very time-consuming and tended to date very quickly. Part of the district's development plan was the establishment of CMHTs, one for North Southwark and three in Lewisham. In the event, only two teams for Lewisham were appointed. The hospital residents were then assigned to a CMHT according to their admission address, and it was the team's responsibility to assess and rehouse the residents.

In West Lambeth, the CMHT was already fully occupied with providing services to the community, and so a separate four-member high support team was established by late 1986, which was to be funded for three years by the Special Trustees of St Thomas's, to assess residents and help them make the transition to the community.

With so many staff involved in assessment, most districts saw the need to systematize the assessment process. Some of the CMHTs in Lewisham and North Southwark used *Getting to Know You* (devised by the Campaign for the Mentally Handicapped (CMH) 1982) as a basis for collecting information. The West Lambeth high support team used *Pathways to Independence* (1982) devised by Jeffrae and Cheseldine, as an initial procedure. In all cases, they added considerable personal knowledge of their residents.

Camberwell had suffered from a series of management problems, but a newly appointed consultant began by undertaking reviews of each resident, calling in CMHT members to help assess mobility and other skills. The CMHT thus gradually got drawn into the assessment of the Darenth Park residents, although their initial brief was to confine their attention to the needs for community services. The appointment of support workers and house managers several months in advance of the opening of houses involved another group of staff with assessment and the grouping process. Finally, at the end of 1986, a resettlement officer was appointed to take charge of the process.

Forming groups among the residents
The overwhelming majority of Darenth Park residents were to live in groups rather than in individual placements, and the purpose of the assessments was to identify compatible groups as well as the service needs of individuals.

All of the districts decided people would not be grouped according to levels of ability because this would scarcely be seen as creating a 'normal' environment, both for the residents and their neighbours. Such a grouping would only result in a houseful of people with the same weaknesses and shortages of skills, something that would not foster good relationships within the house. Likewise, neighbours would tend to view all mentally handicapped people as 'the same', particularly those with greater disabilities. Instead, the principal criterion for grouping residents was friendship. Residents were asked with whom they would like to live and the districts tried, as far as possible, to ensure that these preferences were met. In some instances, this meant 'swapping' residents between different sectors to allow friends to live together.

What districts found, however, was that the majority of residents did not have strong preferences, and so they were compelled to try and create compatible groups. This was carried out on the basis of common interests, compatibility in terms of behaviour, life-style and personalities (e.g. not grouping boisterous and noisy people with elderly residents), avoiding known incompatibilities, and taking account of geographical preferences. Many of the staff interviewed found this the hardest part of their work, because they had to make decisions about the preferences of people whom they hardly knew. The 'getting to know' stage had by its very nature to occur over time because many residents would only begin to express their preferences or wishes after they began to trust the new staff. Through visiting the hospital, district staff were able to spend time with groups of residents either in the hospital's training facilities, or in empty wards which were given to districts to use as a meeting place, or by taking the residents out of the hospital to see how various combinations of people got on together. In some districts, the views of the nursing staff were sought as to how compatible groups of residents were. In other districts, nursing staff were thought to be too judgemental or protective of residents and their views were not specifically sought. The grouping of residents was in no case treated as a paper exercise. Support workers for the houses were allowed in most cases a final say in the groupings.

Some districts had more difficulty in forming groups than others. In West Lambeth, only 30 residents were to transfer to the district, and this small number gave little flexibility to groups formation. In Bromley, there was if anything too much choice: the district was taking 152 residents. It had a purpose-built hostel of three 8-place units, a 72-place residential centre of nine houses (having a maximum of eight residents each), and places available in an existing hostel which was originally intended for women only. Changes were frequently made to lists of groups to meet the following conditions:

● ground floor accommodation for those in wheelchairs or unable to walk stairs;
● keeping friends together;
● keeping a balance of the sexes within groups;
● allowing those wanting a single bedroom to have one;
● introducing men into the all-women's hostel;
● ensuring groups were at least compatible – if not based on friendship, in terms of conversational ability and behaviour.

However much thought is given to groupings of residents, it seems inevitable that some residents will be assigned to a group of their own merely by being rejected by others: they may have no known friendships, or they may present with disruptive or unsociable behaviour which is thought harmful or unpleasant to others. These residents are different from those who simply have no known friendships but who can be brought into groups on a slightly random basis. Some districts have met this problem by designating one facility for those with 'challenging' behaviour, whether officially or otherwise. Other similar residents have been accepted by the special development team and have services and accommodation designed specifically for them.

All districts were involved in 'swapping' residents as a way of maintaining identified friendships. In most cases, this happened during assessment before the residents moved out, but occasionally it occurred after one of the residents had moved out and had expressed his or her unhappiness at a missed friend. Other exchanges were made because parents or relatives had moved to another district and wanted their family member near them. Usually, such exchanges were made easily, although in one or two cases financial considerations may have thwarted an exchange, e.g. if a district was giving up a very able resident for one who was more severely handicapped.

Individual placements

The Region's funding policy had been posited on the assumption that some residents would be placed in the community at little or no cost to a district and these 'savings' would be used to balance out the cost of more intense services. Only one district, Dartford and Gravesham, has made a special arrangement to find places in the private and voluntary sectors. In other districts, private and voluntary places were the outcome of the assessment process which decided what sort of arrangements would be best for particular residents. Such placements were made for specific reasons:

- a wish to be near a relative;
- a requirement for a specialist facility such as psychiatric services or a nursing home;
- a wish to remain in the Dartford area;
- a wish to return to an area of origin.

Liaison took place with local social workers about choosing places in hostels or Part III accommodation if this was seen as appropriate. In at least two cases, districts have paid the cost of additional staff to ensure that their residents got the services they required.

Only six residents returned to live with relatives, and in each case this was because the relation – usually a brother or a sister – wanted this to be so.

Preparing individuals to move

Care staff were appointed in advance of the facilities opening in order to get to know the residents and help them prepare for their move. The hospital helped by making some facilities available where staff and clients could spend time together.

Clients met with staff as individuals and as a group, to see how they got on together. They began by staying in the hospital as a group, having a cup of tea or perhaps preparing a snack or light meal together. They were able to visit the local shops, pubs, outdoor market, pedestrian shopping precinct, libraries, cafés, cinema or bingo hall in the Dartford area, individually or in a group. They visited friends in other wards or other training centres. Sometimes special outings were arranged to London.

In helping to prepare clients for their move, staff would help them to identify the kinds of activities they enjoyed doing or would like to try, the kinds of food they especially enjoyed, what personal possessions they would take with them from Darenth Park, and what sorts of things they would like in their new homes. The clients were taken to see their new homes, even if the builders were still working on them. Later, before the final move from Darenth Park, clients were invited to visit their home, have a meal, stay overnight and then for a weekend, so that they could familiarize themselves with the place. In some instances, clients were able to choose personal items such as sheets and towels or furniture for their bedrooms. Staff often encouraged residents to make up an address book and/or photo album of friends from Darenth Park, thus showing them that their life in the hospital had been valued.

Districts were in general very keen to help clients maintain contact with their families. One district, Greenwich, appointed a liaison officer to inform families of what was happening, give them time to express their views and give reassurance when needed. Family members were invited to visit homes before residents moved in, so that they could assess the accommodation for themselves. Many families had, at the beginning of the Darenth Park Project, expressed concern regarding the ability of their hospitalized relative to live in the community, or of the community to tolerate people with a mental handicap living in their midst. The hospital staff, who were the only people the families knew, had little idea of what would happen to residents, and so could offer little comfort or knowledge. However, district staff, especially those who would be working in the homes, were able to allay many of the relatives' fears. In one instance, parents wrote to the Prime Minister because they were so unhappy with their son's placement. They had moved to a neighbouring borough, and the DHA did not have a service suitable for their son, which meant that he could not live as close to them as they would have liked. Yet they too came to accept the placement.

Many other undertakings had to be made before the residents moved out: bank accounts needed to be transferred from the hospital to the local Girobank or building society; residents needed to be registered with GPs; benefits had to be sorted out; medical records had to be transferred; and so on. It was not an easy task to prepare the residents for such a move yet it is a tribute to the direct care staff that in so many cases it went so smoothly that afterwards it was no longer possible to remember the apprehension which surrounded it.

In brief

This chapter illustrates how complex and time-consuming it has been to make the organizational change from a five-sector hospital to small groups of residents living in the community. It has also illustrated how different solutions require action at many different levels of organization – region, district, hospital, support workers.

The most obvious lesson to be learned is the importance of sorting out residents' assignments to districts rapidly, both as a means of assuring residents and their families that they will be looked after, and as a way of helping districts get on with the task of preparing the facilities. A further important lesson is that of having clearly assigned roles for staff to assess and group residents. It is helpful to have a core of staff who know most, if not all, residents and who have an overview of the services required. Residents, like the rest of us, may want to change their friends and living arrangements, and the staff have to be ready to enable this to happen.

CHAPTER 8

Managing the closure

Achieving a smooth transition

Understandably, public and parliamentary attention has focused on the task of building up adequate alternative services to cater for the existing residents in hospitals that are faced with closure. This was the primary concern of the recent and critical Audit Commission Report (1986). It was also the burden of much discussion in the earlier House of Commons Social Services Committee Report (1985) and its recommendations. For example, Paragraph 40 included what was perhaps the most quoted sentence in the whole report: 'Any fool can close a long stay hospital: it takes more time to do it properly and compassionately.' What the Darenth Park experience demonstrates is that any fool cannot close a hospital that easily – humanely or otherwise. The task of managing closure is at least as complex as opening new facilities. Indeed, it requires even more managerial expertise and flexibility because the pace of closure is dependent on the success and timing of a large number of other schemes that are the responsibility of numerous local district health authorities, social services departments, housing departments and voluntary organizations. In short, the difficulties of achieving closure, without further worsening the quality of life of existing residents, have been underestimated.

To close a long-stay institution 'properly and compassionately' involves achieving several different objectives at the same time:

1 Phasing the contraction of the hospital to coincide with the build up of district-based and community services.
2 Making effective use of remaining staff and saving on running costs.
3 Minimizing the disruption caused by the change in residents' wards and training units and sustaining the quality of their care.
4 Providing satisfactory alternative employment for existing staff, including retraining those who wish to continue to care for mentally handicapped people in new settings.
5 Achieving closure by the planned date to free the capital resources tied up in the site, and financing rundown.

These objectives were identified by the Darenth Park Steering Group in its early discussions. What few foresaw was just how difficult they would be to achieve.

Phasing contraction and alternative service provision

As a means of achieving this objective, the management of the Darenth Park Hospital produced regular annual 'reduction control plans'. The first was published in April 1984. These plans were attempts to estimate the rate of withdrawal of residents as they moved into alternative accommodation and were based on the managers' knowledge of the development plans of the *seven* health districts which used the hospital and the timing assumed in them.

There have been three control plans, in 1984, 1985 and 1986. Each had to be revised in the light of what actually happened in the previous year. Originally, in 1984, it was expected that the number of planned discharges would build up gradually from 58 in 1983 to 248 in 1987–8 (see Table 8.1). Then, as District plans advanced, a faster rate of reprovision was estimated for 1984–5, altering the number who were to leave in the final year to 200, rather than 248. (The proposed bed losses did not always match the

Table 8.1 Planned reductions in numbers of residents

1984 plan	1.4.83	1.4.84	1.4.85	1.4.86	1.4.87	
Planned number of residents	724 (actual)	666	562	401	248	
Proposed discharges during year plus assumed deaths	−58	−104	−182	−174	−248	
1985 plan		1.4.84	1.4.85	1.4.86	1.4.87	
Planned number of residents		689 (actual)	565	328	199	
Proposed discharges during year		−130	−237	−129	−199	
1986 plan			1.4.85	1.4.86	1.4.87	
Planned number of residents			586 (actual)	450 (actual)	184	
Proposed discharges			−266	−196	−184	
					1.4.87	1.4.88
					312 (actual)	118 (actual)

Table 8.2 The pace of discharge 1983–9 (numbers discharged)

	1983–4	*1984–5*	*1985–6*	*1986–7*	*1987–8*	*1988–9*
Deaths	20	27	27	23	8	—
Discharge to replacement NHS facilities	18	49	116	85	186	105
Miscellaneous discharges	23	22	22	13	25	13
Total	61	98	165	122	219	118

Table 8.3 Residents remaining in the hospital on the last day of each month, 1978–89

Year	*April*	*May*	*June*	*July*	*Aug.*	*Sept.*	*Oct.*	*Nov.*	*Dec.*	*Jan.*	*Feb.*	*March*
1978–9	993	990	991	991	997	993	980	976	973	973	971	961
1979–80	956	953	953	952	947	947	943	943	938	936	930	914
1980–81	912	910	903	899	878	871	863	861	861	853	849	846
1981–2	847	841	840	832	822	817	816	814	806	797	783	776
1982–3	776	760	754	752	749	747	737	731	730	728	720	716
1983–4	708	704	705	703	703	699	695	688	683	681	679	677
1984–5	675	673	671	667	660	643	622	615	616	615	605	583
1985–6	576	559	557	553	553	554	549	545	529	471	469	450
1986–7	441	435	422	414	405	392	384	375	371	359	353	345
1987–8	312	297	270	257	250	240	235	214	206	202	184	125
1988–9	118	105	75	41								

discharges because some delay was expected in terms of the phased opening of new developments.)

By April 1986, however, serious slippage had occurred so that there were still 450 residents rather than the planned figure of 328. Of the 203 discharges planned for the previous financial year, only 116 actually took place, 22 of which were to existing facilities, which meant many more residents would have to be discharged in 1986–7 to get back to the original target. This did not happen, and when the proposed closure date of 31 March 1988 was reached, 118 residents remained in Darenth Park, requiring the hospital to stay open for a further 4½ months (see Tables 8.2 and 8.3).

Reasons for the delay

1 *Capital schemes fell behind schedule.* All districts experienced delays, in some cases quite serious ones, in the building or conversion of accommodation: building schemes took longer than at first thought; some firms went bankrupt; new tenders were needed; and several conversion schemes

also took longer than planned. In retrospect, it would seem wise for planners to allow for delays of this kind.

2 *Unsatisfactory original design specifications caused losses.* We have already discussed Archery House, the main residential facility for Dartford and Gravesham, which was designed for 96 residents. When staff came to inspect the completed facility, they realized that it would be impossible to fit the furniture, residents and wheelchairs into the space available. It took 6 months to secure the agreement of the health authority to reduce the number of residents to be housed from 96 to 80. Other districts also experienced design faults resulting in additional unplanned building work.

3 *Changing district plans.* Another difficulty faced by the hospital managers was that districts' plans changed as they changed their ideas about the kind of services they would provide.

4 *Financial constraints.* These caused some authorities to delay opening facilities that could have been opened on time. The opening of a hostel in Bexley was delayed by 6 months while the district tried to get additional funds from the Region. In Camberwell, the district simply halted its housing programme because it was unable to contribute additional revenue spending to meet the standards required by the Mental Handicap Unit managers.

5 *The opening* of the larger facilities had to be phased to permit residents to move in small numbers. The 72 residents scheduled to go to Bassetts Village in Bromley were transferred over a 4-month period. Further, Bromley Health Authority decided to absorb into Bassetts its 24 residents then living in Grove Park Hospital, leaving more residents in Darenth Park than the hospital managers had anticipated.

6 *Staffing difficulties.* Staff shortages at Darenth Park itself meant that the promised transfer of staff out to the new community facilities in Dartford and Gravesham could not take place, and thus the transfer of residents from the hospital was also delayed. Other districts experienced difficulties in recruiting trained and experienced staff, and this too led to delays.

7 *Unforeseen admissions.* Darenth Park was closed to short-term and long-term admissions from all districts other than Dartford and Gravesham on 1 April 1984. The managing district continued to use Darenth Park for short-term care. However, it had to take seven long-term admissions when a unit at another hospital for both long- and short-stay residents with a mental handicap and mental illness closed. Its closure had originally been planned to coincide with the closure of Darenth Park, its residents being transferred to Dartford's new unit at Archery House. However, this was pre-empted by the need for the unit to be released for geriatric patients transferring from a hospital in Gravesend which was also being closed.

The range of these problems illustrates how difficult it is for reduction control planning to proceed as expected. Regional planners are apt not to be open or explicit about this, in case it reduces the pressure on districts to

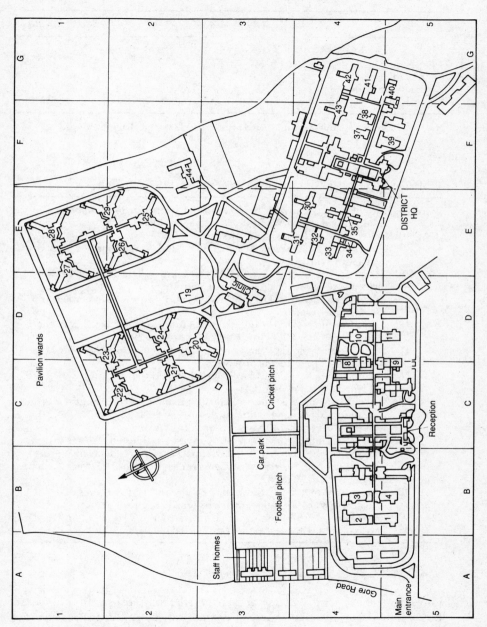

Figure 8.1 Darenth Park Hospital.

Table 8.4 Ward closures 1983–9

	1.4.83	1.4.84	1.4.85	1.4.86	1.4.87	1.4.88
1984 plan	33	32	21	9	—	
1985 plan	33	30	17	12	0	
1986 plan			20	7	0	
Actual number of wards open	37	33	30	20	15	7

Note: These figures exclude the three shared wards (special needs and infirmary wards).

Table 8.5 Ward closures and movement of residents, 1986–7

Ward 8: Closed June, Greenwich/Bexley, North Southwark and Camberwell residents transfer to Ward 40, 3 Bromley residents to Ward 35/6

   40: Reopened June for residents of Ward 8

   5B: Closed July. Camberwell, West Lambeth and North Southwark residents transfer to Ward 29

   28: Temporarily reopened July for Dartford/Gravesham and Camberwell residents, to allow for upgrading of Ward 29

   29: Transferred July from Dartford/Gravesham sector to Camberwell and West Lambeth sector

   28: Closed August; 5 Dartford/Gravesham residents discharged to Archery House, 2 transfer to Ward 29, 2 Camberwell to 29

   41: Closed September to Greenwich/Bexley residents who transfer to Ward 25, reopened to residents of Ward 6

    6: Closed September; Camberwell/West Lambeth/North Southwark residents transfer to Ward 41

   5A: Closed September to Camberwell/West Lambeth, North Southwark and non-allocated residents who transfer to Ward 28

   28: Reopened September to residents of Ward 5A

   25: Closed September when Dartford/Gravesham children transfer to another hospital. Reopened to Greenwich/Bexley residents of Ward 41

 35/6: Closed October; 5 Bromley residents transfer to Ward 25, 5 to Ward 21, 1 Greenwich to Ward 43

   30: Closed November; 5 Greenwich, 2 Bexley and 1 Bromley resident transfer to Ward 28, 1 Greenwich to Ward 26, 2 to Ward 25

   33: Closed February; 4 Bromley residents transfer to Ward 23, 3 to Ward 22, 2 to Ward 20, 1 Bexley resident to Ward 42

implement change and encourages further delays. Realistically, however, hospital managers must take these problems into account so as to ensure that their own plans are not thrown into disarray. The Regional officers, who kept Darenth Park informed of the districts' plans, tended to be over-optimistic as regards the ability of the districts to keep to their plans.

Minimizing disruption to residents

Ward closures

The rate at which residents were transferred to districts affected the ward closure programme. Hospital managers had several objectives which needed to be balanced in achieving the physical contraction of the hospital: minimizing disruption to the residents; making effective use of the remaining staff; saving on the running costs of the hospital; closing the most unsuitable wards; helping districts to bring together residents who would be living together in the community; and keeping those staff and residents who knew each other together as far as possible.

Figure 8.1 shows the distribution of hospital buildings on site. The overall scheme was for the hospital to contract towards the pavilion wards away from the main buildings, thus making the greatest possible savings on services (e.g. heating) and retaining the maximum amount of ground-floor accommodation. Each pavilion ward was able to accommodate about 24 residents (see Table 8.4 for the planned and actual closure of wards at Darenth Park). In practice, however, the scheme was not as straightforward as it sounds. Besides the movement necessary to concentrate residents within the pavilion sites, a number of wards were closed and then reopened. The movements, closures and reopenings undertaken in just one year, 1986–7, are shown in Table 8.5; Table 8.6 shows movements in and out of wards during the last 20 months the hospital was open.

In 1986–7, residents in 14 out of the 20 wards remaining open experienced major disruptions associated with being moved from one ward to another. It is inherent in any closure programme that such disruption occurs. These planned movements were exacerbated by the age and dilapidation of the buildings and the desire to use ground floor accommodation where possible, and the additional workloads placed on nursing and portering staff should not be underestimated.

Residents' changes of wards

Of the 650 or so residents discharged from the hospital since 1983 (excluding deaths), 65% experienced no more than one move before discharge (the stated aim). Table 8.7 shows how this varied between the districts. The Dartford and Gravesham residents came off the best, with 85% having faced no more than one move and only 3% experiencing three or more moves. Camberwell and Bromley came off worst: 50 and 55%, respectively, having made no more than one move; 20 and 23%, respectively, experiencing three or more moves. Dartford and Gravesham had its five wards in the pavilion from the start, and therefore their residents hardly needed to move at all. The Camberwell and Bromley residents were affected by the first ward clsoures at the end of 1983, and by many of the ensuing ward closure programmes.

Table 8.6 Ward movements: change of wards by residents

Ward	1987									1988							
	Apr.	May	June	July	Aug.	Sept.	Oct.	Nov.	Dec.	Jan.	Feb.	Mar.	Apr.	May	June	July	Aug.
19	-1 Res.	-2										-2	-1	-2	+3 -3	-4	
20	+6 -3	-1		+9 -10	-3		-1	-2	-2			-7	+9	-2	-6	-5	
21				-1	-1	-1 +2	-2	-2	-2			+4 -4	-1		closed -7		
22	+7 -6	-1		-4	-2	+8		-4	-2	-3		closed -9					
23		-3		-3	-1	+3					-2	closed -1					
24			-1	-3		+5 -1		-1	-1	-2	-2	-11	+3 -2	-1	+5 -3	-7	
25	+4 -2		-6	+1 -3	closed -1	reopens +24 -2		-1					-2	-1	-2	-6	
26								-3	-1	-1	-1	-5	closed				
27	-1	-3	-1	-2				-2	-1	-1	-1	+7 -6	-1 -5	closed			
28	-1	-3		-1		+5		-2	-1	-8	-4	closed			-7		
29	+8					-2		-4	-1		+8 -5		-2	+4 -3			
31	closed -3																
32	closed -12																
40						closed -1											
41						closed -6											
42				closed -1		closed											
43	-2		-3														

Table 8.7 Residents' moves before discharge by district

Borough	No moves	1 move	2 moves	3 or more moves
Bexley	17	12	13	8
Bromley	27	45	32	24
Camberwell	19	37	32	26
Dartford/Gravesham	60	49	15	4
Greenwich	44	35	26	16
Lewisham/N. Southwark	22	32	16	8
West Lambeth	1	16	6	3

It is possible that some of these changes could have been avoided, but this would have meant discharging greater numbers of residents at a time, so that whole wards could be closed. The wards, too, would have had to have been closed in an agreed order. The districts tried both to respect friendships and form compatible house groups, which meant that residents were more likely to be discharged in twos and threes. At the outset, the number of wards was reduced gradually; however, this process was speeded up as the nursing staff contracted, because it became necessary to concentrate the residents in fewer wards so as to ensure their safety.

There was concern too, for the safety of hospital staff, particularly those on night duty. Not only were the wards scattered over the hospital grounds, but security was worsened once demolition began. The management, therefore, needed to ensure that no ward was left isolated as others around it closed.

A natural consequence of these changes was that the number of residents on most wards increased. In April 1983, the 18-bed wards, mainly Wards 1–9, had an average of 11.5 residents; however, their average occupancy increased to 16.8 residents towards the end of 1986 when they finally closed.

The planned ward closures also took place against a background of unplanned ward closures, made necessary by poor conditions or increasingly inadequate services, such as heating and water. During the winter of 1985–6, for example, the floor of a special care unit collapsed and the residents occupying Wards 33, 3A, 3B and 4B had to be moved at short notice to alternative accommodation because of leaks and contamination of the hot water system.

Planning the reduction of staff

In 1983, at the time the first reduction control plan was drawn up, Darenth Park Hospital employed 939 staff, excluding medical and dental staff (WTE of 810.66). A brief profile of the staff is given in Table 8.8. The personnel department hoped that by relying on natural wastage, redeployment and

Table 8.8 Darenth Park Hospital staff in March 1983

Male	27.1% (252)
Female	72.9% (677)
Part-time	35.2%
Full-time	64.8% (males 94.8%; females 53.7%)

Age
under 21	89 (9.5%)
21–30	181 (19.3%)
31–40	242 (25.8%)
41–50	223 (23.8%)
51–60	165 (17.6%)
61–65	38 (4.0%)
65+	1 (0.1%)

Years worked at Darenth Park Hospital
under 2	219 (23.3%)
2–5	277 (29.5%)
6–10	250 (26.6%)
11–15	112 (12.0%)
16–20	48 (5.1%)
21+	33 (3.5%)

Note: 939 staff equivalent to 810.66 WTE

redundancies would not be necessary. Furthermore, redundancy payments would be limited due to the high number of part-time staff employed. Finally, 57 staff were to reach compulsory retirement age and a further 92 would be of an age to take voluntary retirement (60 years for women and 55 for nurses) by the time the hospital closed.

The 1984 reduction control plan was drawn up shortly after the appointment of two reduction control personnel officers, one responsible for the nursing staff and the other for the non-nursing staff. This initial attempt at forecasting staff reductions (and all subsequent plans) was based on the following assumptions:

● The standard of residential care would be of the same quality.
● Staffing levels would not be reduced pro rata with the number of residents discharged. Indeed, staffing ratios would need to be increased due to the turbulence that closure would cause and the tendency for districts to transfer the less dependent residents first.

The planned loss of about 44 staff in 1983–4 was achieved by natural wastage. In 1984–5, however, two staff were made compulsorily redundant: one for health reasons, the other because he could not be redeployed. Despite the redundancies, the number of staff employed at the end of the financial year was 43 below the target level of 728. The overall staff was short by 6 caterers, 10 domestics and 48 qualified nurses.

The hospital's major concern was to retain an adequate nursing staff. The shortfall in the number of qualified nurses was relieved in a number of ways: the hospital employed a larger number of nursing assistants; the existing nursing staff were allowed to work overtime; a number of qualified nurses were employed through agencies; and a nurse bank scheme was created with a local job centre. This latter scheme attracted a number of nurses who had retired and some who were 'moonlighting' from other hospitals and who were willing to do an extra 2 or 3 shifts a week. By working the same shifts each week, they were able to get to know the residents and be counted as part of the nursing team. The bank scheme began in March 1985, when overtime and agency staff were already contributing the equivalent of between an extra 15 and 20 staff monthly. The cost of these schemes presented no problems, because the nursing budget was underspent. Despite frequent reminders that the hospital was short of nursing staff and conditions were critical, hospital management seemed to manage the situation reasonably well. Qualified nurses represented 39% of the total nursing staff in April 1984, a figure that was slightly improved upon in the following years (see Table 8.9).

In general, hospital management tried to keep a balance between staffing levels and the safety of the residents. What perhaps was given less thought was the maintenance of an adequate level of recreational and entertainment activities: in the second year of the reduction control plan, the manager of the Pets' Corner and the recreations officer both left. These two posts both represented opportunities for activities off the wards. In hindsight, it would seem that funds should have been kept to ensure that a full range of activities are available up to the time of closure.

Redeployment of staff

The first step in planning redeployment is to find out what the intentions of the staff are. In 1984, the reduction control personnel officers interviewed each staff member individually to ascertain what their future employment plans were. By discussing anything that might influence their employment potential (e.g. whether they owned a car or had family commitments), management were able to create an overall picture of each member of staff. The outcome of these interviews was as follows:

- 275 staff wished to work at Archery House;
- 161 wished to work with the mentally handicapped in community housing in Dartford and Gravesham;
- 275 wanted to stay at Darenth Park until it was closed;
- 231 would accept similar employment within Dartford and Gravesham;
- 78 would consider any other work within Dartford and Gravesham;
- 9 non-nursing staff were willing to work elsewhere in Kent;
- 18 were prepared to travel to London; and
- 65 were willing to travel to Bromley or Bexley.

Table 8.9 Staffing at Darenth Park 1985–8

	Qualified nursing staff as a percentage of all nursing staff	
	Qualified nurses (%)	Qualified nurses (including overtime, agency, bank staff) (%)
April 1985	38.7	41.5
April 1986	37.9	43.5
April 1987	39.3	42.6
April 1988	40.0	43.8
	Resident-Staffing rations	
	Staff : resident (Darenth staff only)[a]	Staff : resident (including overtime, etc.)
April 1984	1 : 1.6	—
April 1985	1 : 1.7	1 : 1.6
April 1986	1 : 1.7	1 : 1.7
April 1987	1 : 1.6	1 : 1.2
April 1988	1 : 0.88	1 : 0.64

[a] No allowance is made for those staff working nights only, or absence/sickness leave; includes all nursing staff.

It became obvious that the cooperation of other districts would be necessary if a significant number of redundancies was to be avoided.

In August 1984, a meeting of the district personnel officers within the hospital's catchment area was arranged to facilitate the redeployment of staff and enlist the aid of other districts in maintaining adequate staffing levels at Darenth Park until its closure. Two factors worked against those staff transferring to other districts, however. First, Darenth Park was on the edge of the catchment area, and therefore staff would face long (and expensive) journeys to work in inner London. Perhaps more significantly, the inner-London districts were very different in character from Dartford, both socially and politically. Those staff who had lived and worked in the Dartford area for many years were reluctant to move. Neither were the receiving districts always very keen to cooperate. Initially, they felt that it was right to handpick their employees and that staff from Darenth Park would not be able to work in the new non-hospital services.

As has already been stated, the hospital's main concern was with the loss of qualified nurses. The director of nursing services (DNS) at Darenth Park was eager for other districts to offer these nurses employment in the new services, provided they stayed at Darenth Park until all of the residents they were responsible for left. However, the DNS felt that few nurses would take up employment in other districts while positions within Dartford's new services remained unfilled. Therefore, it was agreed that Dartford would recruit for Archery House and its staffed group homes before the other districts could interview Darenth Park staff.

However, new difficulties soon became apparent. Three districts had a non-nursing staffing structure which prevented them from paying qualified nurses on nursing salary scales to care for residents in the new settings. Any nurse transferring to one of these districts would have to give up their mental health nursing officer status and the right to early retirement. In addition, several districts were closing hospitals within their own boundaries, and their personnel officers were naturally inclined to give priority to staff already employed within those districts.

The personnel officers faced several additional problems in trying to redeploy staff. Many staff did not believe that the hospital would ever close: it might get – and was getting – smaller, but it would never close completely. With this in mind, the hospital managers were keen to demolish some closed wards, simply to indicate to staff that change was on the way. In late 1984, the first two ward blocks to close were demolished, as was another ward near the District's headquarters. The Steering Group intentionally held its meeting at Darenth Park to witness the demolition and had a small celebration. This angered many staff, who claimed it was wrong to celebrate the demolition of people's homes. Darenth Park *was* home to its residents, but the staff were also protesting about the intrusion of reality into their wishful thinking.

For some staff, it had been many years since they had applied for jobs, and so they needed help in filling out application forms, and coaching on how to present themselves in interviews. The personnel department organized training days for staff to help them understand the process better, and conducted mock interviews. They found that this counselling placed great demands on their time.

The personnel officers also had to face the fact that service managers had failed in their personnel duties on a number of occasions. There were several instances where staff had been kept on when they should have been retired on the grounds of ill-health. In some departments, serious absenteeism was not followed up by management, and managers in other services were not keen to employ such people. In such cases, there was little the personnel department could do. Also, over the years, a number of employees were redeployed to Darenth Park because other district services did not want them.

Many staff seemed prepared to 'sit it out', hoping to take redundancy payments at the time the hospital closed, and would then be free to take on other jobs unless they retired. As a means of countering this, the Mental Handicap Unit Management Group in Dartford sent a letter to all staff at the hospital in September 1985, outlining the personnel rundown procedures. Three different approaches were identified according to whether departments had more, fewer or an adequate number of staff in relation to the reduction control plan target for that year; in each case, the principle was last in, first out (LIFO). At the beginning of each financial year, redundancy notices would be issued to employees in those departments which were over-staffed, according to the final staff target for that year. The notices would be issued to those staff who joined that department last; if vacancies in similar departments became available in other hospitals within the district, those staff employed longest in the department would be offered them, and the redundancy notice would be withdrawn. In those departments where there was the right number of staff or fewer staff than were needed, staff would be encouraged to apply for alternative employment in Dartford or the other districts. Those staff successful in finding alternative employment would be issued with new contracts, even if they remained at Darenth Park for a while. Salaries would be protected if staff in departments with excess numbers accepted a post on a lower grade; if staff in other departments accepted a post on a lower grade, having refused a post on the same or similar grade, protection would not be automatic.

As part of this process, a 'reservation of posts' scheme was started, with departmental managers identifying those key workers who were most needed at the hospital until its closure. This allowed posts to be reserved for these staff in other hospitals, their positions in the meantime being filled by temporary staff. This scheme resulted in the issuing of more than 100 temporary contracts to staff in the Dartford District.

After April 1988, redundancy notices were handed out more system-atically. On 1 July, 3 months' notice was given to the rehabilitation and administrative and clerical staff (except for identified key workers); from 1 August, notice was given to all temporary domestics (less than 2 years service), temporary porters and the hairdresser. Then, after the hospital closed, notice was given to long-servicing domestics and catering staff.

All of this was predictable and necessary, but it was not realized just how unpleasant it would be. It is intrinsically difficult to tell people that they are no longer needed, even if they have been employed temporarily. It was made even more difficult because the closure of Darenth Park was so drawn out – first it was to be in March, then June, then July, then suddenly August. The longest-serving staff were often the most difficult to deal with. Quite a number of people did not take up the posts that were reserved for them – they simply did not want to move, and were often unable to give a reason why. They resented the hospital closing and were not willing to give the new jobs a go. The hospital had had a very stable core of staff, and no matter how many warnings were given, they refused to move.

A total of 448 staff were redeployed, just about half the number of staff employed at the hospital in 1983. Of this total, 288 (excluding 20 retirements) were nurses, so that 65% of the nursing staff were kept in nursing, in the catchment area the majority of them in mental handicap nursing. Several nursing auxiliaries left to undertake training. In the end, only 7 of the 16 nurses who expressed interest in transferring to Leybourne Grange Hospital did so.

Funding the rundown and achieving closure on time

Under the Region's mental handicap funding policy, Darenth Park Hospital lost the equivalent of the average inpatient expenditure per head for every death and discharge from the hospital in the following financial year. This figure formed the savings target which the hospital should have achieved. The resources available to the hospital were controlled separately from the District's general allocation, the basis of which was the hospital's 1982–3 expenditure out-turn (the time at which the Region's mental handicap funding policy came into operation), which had subsequently been upgraded to reflect annual pay and price increases.

It was recognized that the revenue savings which the hospital could achieve would not be in direct proportion to the reduction in the number of residents, because, for example, those residents who remained demanded a greater level of care. It was the responsibility of Dartford and Gravesham District to inform the Region of the proportion of the savings target which it felt could be achieved by taking such factors into account. Because there was bound to be a process of negotiation between Region and District, a preliminary figure was calculated on an August to July basis to allow negotiations to be completed before the start of the new financial year in the following April. This process ended in 1986, when the savings target was related to discharges in the previous financial year (see Table 8.10).

The District began the negotiating process with a savings target based on deaths and discharges. This sum was then divided into two parts: variable expenditure, which it could afford to lose because of the reduced number of residents, and fixed expenditure, which it could not lose if an adequate level of services was to be maintained for the remaining residents. The District requested bridging finance from the Region for its fixed expenditure, or non-recurring revenue.

Money continued to be spent at Darenth Park after the last residents left the

Table 8.10 Funding the rundown

	Target savings (£)	Savings achieved (£)	Planned discharges (no.)	Actual discharges (no.)
1983–4	570 372	520 000	58	52
1984–5	1 022 736	500 000	130	98
1985–6	2 119 415	1 350 000	237	146
1986–7	2 252 642	1 250 000	266	104
1987–8	5 007 556	2 521 000	184	219
1988–9	2 262 000		118	118

Note: The total of planned discharges does not equal the total of actual discharges because planned discharges are taken from different prediction control plans, as plans of districts changed. The important point is that between 1983–4 and 1987–8, actual discharges always fell short of planned discharges.

hospital. There were, for example, expenses associated with providing temporary facilities at Stone House and Truscott Villas. There were also expenses associated with closing down Darenth Park buildings – making them secure, removing furniture and administrative records of various kinds, closing down services – costs which could be negotiated separately with the Region. In each year, the District was successful in convincing the Region to reduce the amount of revenue to be handed back because actual discharges did not match planned discharges. The Region's main concern was that Darenth Park was not 'overfunded', money that could be channelled into other district services. In addition to the revenue support, capital support was also given for the maintenance activities associated with ward changes and closures (making buildings no longer being used secure and safe, e.g. removing asbestos), and revenue support for staff training. The training budget was initially £7500 p.a. for 4 years, starting in 1982–3; in fact, it was scarcely used in the first year, and the hospital was successful in getting this fund extended for a further year.

Departure day

On 1 August 1988, 41 residents remained in Darenth Park, 15 of whom were discharged to their districts between 5 and 11 August, leaving 26 residents on the last day. To close the hospital by the agreed date, the hospital manager had to transfer residents to a ward at Stone House Hospital, a mental illness hospital next to Archery House, and to two villas intended for residents from Stone House who were not yet ready to be discharged.

The move to Stone House Hospital went well, but the move to the villas was less smooth. Because the principal administrator at Darenth Park was on holiday just before the hospital closed, the work of preparing the villas had not been completed on time, and the residents and staff arrived to find beds unmade and an inadequate supply of crockery and other items. These were put right immediately, but it was an unfortunate ending to the closure process.

The 20 residents who were temporarily taken on by Dartford belonged to Greenwich, Bexley and Camberwell Health Authorities. The one Bexley resident and the five Greenwich residents stayed for 2 weeks, until the end of August. Six Camberwell residents transferred back to their district at the end of September; one other was placed temporarily in a staffed group home in Dartford. This allowed the two villas to close. Five men – four from Camberwell and one from Greenwich – remained on their own male ward in Stone House at the end of 1988. One woman, originating from Brighton and intending to return there as soon as a place was found for her, remained on a ward by herself.

After closure

Once the last resident left Darenth Park, considerable work remained to be done. The wards needed to be cleared of furniture, though the administration abandoned an inventory system because so much was damaged and some things just went missing. The buildings were extremely difficult to make secure. The three-storey ward blocks by the hospital entrance, which had been built on sloping ground, had their windows at different levels in different parts of the building. Even after bricking up all of the ground-floor windows, it was still possible to enter the buildings. Making them truly secure would have probably cost more than demolishing them.

The remaining furniture and equipment was offered to other services and districts, while the administrative records were sorted and stored or destroyed. The services needed for the District headquarters, due to remain on site for a further 2–4 years, were identified (gardening, catering and cleaning), and separate budgets created. Other buildings on the site were also closed, and the nurses' residence was being considered for rent to the local council. The riding school has remained, and the laundry was still open in 1989 supplying other hospitals.

As for the 200-acre site, part of it is wanted by the District for a new headquarters, allowing the rationalization of smaller acute units. An application for selling part of the land for housing has been sent to the Secretary of State for the Environment.

In brief

The complexity of, and the human problems involved in, closing an institution the size of Darenth Park were underestimated from the beginning. Plans were subject to much more uncertainty than was ever envisaged. Managers had to devise coping strategies right up to the last moment. The central lesson to be learned is that top-class managerial skills are required to achieve this apparently unglamorous task. It is to be hoped that senior management in other regions and districts will learn this lesson. Darenth Park Hospital was fortunate to have the management that it did, for without them the closure could have turned into a disaster.

PART 3

An evaluation

CHAPTER 9

New homes, new lives

In Chapter 7 we described some of the characteristics of the residents who were in Darenth Park in 1980, as assessed by Dr Lorna Wing. Eight years later, when the hospital had closed and the residents were distributed among seven districts, some changes in these characteristics have occurred. Of the approximately 650 residents discharged to places identified by districts, there was a marked increase in the percentage of the population as a whole who were aged 80 or over – 8% in 1988 as opposed to 4.1% in 1980. Since 1980, 194 residents had died, resulting in a marginal increase in the number of men over women; in two districts, however, this imbalance was noticeably greater. The number of residents assessed as totally dependent on wheelchairs had fallen from 122 to 75, although there is likely to be an increase in the number of wheelchair-bound residents as the population ages – this will become known through Wing's follow-up assessments. A slight shift towards a larger percentage of residents who are socially impaired has occurred (see Tables 9.1 and 9.2). This is the status of the residents whose futures were planned by their districts.

Before 1983, the pattern had been different. Most departures followed the more-or-less usual pattern of hospital discharges, arranged by consultant and nursing staff: some went home, some went to live in bed-and-breakfast accommodation in seaside hotels. The one exception was the opening of The Gables Hostel in Greenwich in 1982, which took 30 residents from Darenth Park.

Table 9.3 shows how the pattern changed and also helps to demonstrate that regional officers were right to accept that Darenth Park would not close on time if they relied on purpose-built facilities to be developed for all residents. Two new hostels opened in 1984 and 1985 in Bromley and Greenwich. Archery House received its first residents in January 1986, Bassetts Village in April 1987 and Bowley Close in Camberwell in March 1988. Planning for all these projects had begun in 1978 and 1979.

In contrast, the first two group homes, identified in 1982, were opened in Camberwell in April 1983 and in Dartford in November 1983. The districts began planning for many group homes in 1984, and 8 opened in 1985–6, 7 in

Table 9.1 Age of residents in 1988

Age	Bexley	Bromley	Camberwell	Dartford/ Gravesham	Greenwich	Lewisham/ North Southwark	West Lambeth	Total (No.)	(%)
0–9	—	—	—	—	—	—	—	—	—
10–19	—	—	1	—	—	—	—	1	(0.2)
20–29	9	1	12	21	5	5	—	53	(8.2)
30–39	15	20	26	22	31	21	3	138	(21.3)
40–49	14	13	18	22	16	14	3	100	(15.5)
50–59	6	14	14	24	20	9	1	88	(13.6)
60–69	5	29	20	20	23	13	10	120	(18.5)
70–79	2	30	15	14	19	11	4	95	(14.7)
80–89	—	19	6	6	8	6	4	49	(7.6)
90+	—	1	2	—	—	—	1	4	(0.5)
Male	31	64	72	78	72	45	15	377	(58.2)
Female	20	63	42	51	50	34	11	271	(41.8)

Table 9.2 Physical and sensory handicaps of residents in 1980 (clients discharged to districts only)

	Bexley	Bromley	Camberwell	Dartford/Gravesham	Greenwich	Lewisham/North Southwark	West Lambeth
Wheelchair-bound	7	10	17	25	6	9	1
Blind	—	.2	1	9	4	4	2
Deaf	—	—	1	—	1	—	—
Blind and deaf	—	—	2	1	2	1	—
Behaviour characteristics							
1	19	23	32	25	28	17	2
2	9	19	19	36	19	12	2
3	6	24	11	11	21	18	7
4	12	53	42	47	50	29	15
Not assessed	5	8	10	10	4	3	—

Table 9.3 Place of discharge

	78/79	79/80	80/81	81/82	82/83	83/84	84/85	85/86	86/87	87/88	88/89	Total
Death	41	29	33	30	33	20	27	25	18	8	—	264
Self-discharge	6	3	2	4	—	—	1	1	1	1	—	17
Home (1)	6	4	1	3	3	3	1	2	1	—	—	24
Seaside town	8	12	5	4	3	—	1	3	—	4	—	40
Boarding out (2)	1	1	—	—	2	—	2	1	1	2	—	10
Private home	2	6	4	—	1	2	3	—	4	7	4	33
Vol. home	1	—	—	1	—	2	2	1	3	2 (7)	1	13
Council flat	2	2	1	1	2	—	—	—	1	—	—	9
LA MH hostel	3	—	2	1	2	—	4	—	2	1	—	14
LA OPH/MI hostel	1	1	1	4	5	1	—	—	—	3 (3)	1	17
Other MH hospital	2	2	—	1	1	—	3	1	—	1	1	12
Other hospital	1	2	2	—	1	—	2	—	—	7 (4)	6 (4)	19
Grove Park	1	1	31	24	16	4	2	3	3	4	—	89
NHS hostel	—	2	—	20	11	5	45	23	29	22 (5)	2	159
NHS Residential Centre	—	—	—	—	—	—	—	58	24	92	14	188
Staffed Group home	—	—	—	—	—	14	7	28	17	50	33	149
Training/interim (9)	—	—	—	—	—	—	—	—	—	15	57	72
Miscellaneous (8)	2	—	1	2	2	1	1	—	—	—	—	–9
Total	77	65	82	94	82	52	98	146	104	219	119	1138

Notes
(1) includes parents, sisters, brothers, aunts/uncles
(2) usually private landladies within district or SSD Adult Placement
(3) includes 1 sheltered flat for elderly
(4) includes 4 discharges to MIETS
(5) includes 1 place in Hounslow DHA
(6) includes 1 place in MIETS and 4 in a private hospital
(7) includes a sheltered flat run by a voluntary organization
(8) *Miscellaneous*
78/9 — addresses not identifiable
80/1 — addresses not identifiable
81/2 — residential schools
    — 1 address not identifiable
    — prison
    — emigration to Australia
Interim/training facilities
1988/89 interim/training facilities includes 37 interim places in the receiving districts and 20 interim places in Dartford provided when the hospital closed. Of those, 6 transferred to their remaining districts within two weeks, and by the end of September.

1986–7, 18 in 1987–8 and 13 between April and August 1988 (in addition, several temporary home-type facilities were opened to allow Darenth Park to close). It was felt that even those homes which required considerable renovation would be completed faster than relying on the NHS's own building and capital control system.

About 25% of the residents died in hospital. The assumption by Regional officers that about 30 residents would die each year, thereby reducing the number of places needed in the community, proved to be correct. Self-discharge included those people who did not return to the hospital while on leave or people discharged to 'no fixed abode'. Some residents returned to the hospital, and were then again discharged to the care of a district.

The number of addresses on the discharge lists in places like Ramsgate, Margate and Westgate was actually quite limited, and it was obvious that only a few boarding houses were being used. Several of these were owned or being run by former Darenth Park staff, and residents often went to live in one because they knew the landlady and the other residents. Though these were often initially successful placements, there were a number of problems, e.g. an absence of day activities, additional demands made on the health and social services in these areas without additional funding being provided; there were problems when either a landlady retired or boarding houses were sold. Since 1983–4, when the districts began to take responsibility for former Darenth Park residents, transfer to the care of private and voluntary establishments has been based largely on the availability of specialized services or the close proximity of family members who have moved from the resident's district of origin.

Mention was made in Chapter 6 of the transfer of 43 residents in Greenwich to the care of the social services department. In addition, other local authorities accepted the placement of residents in mental handicap hostels, mental illness hostels or old peoples' homes (Table 9.4 lists the establishments and local authorities involved). Residents who were boarding-out, in adult placement or family placement schemes have also been transferred to the care of the social services.

Where a resident is discharged to is not necessarily, of course, the same place in which a resident is to remain. For example, some placements did not work out as people did not get on together, and some residents decided for other reasons they wanted to live elsewhere. Bromley Health Authority transferred the first group of residents using a hostel to minimally staffed group homes after they received training in the hostels. Other residents in all authorities were able to move to more independent facilities when they were able to show that they were able to cope.

Table 9.5 shows the net changes which have taken place between the time the residents were discharged and where they were living in September 1988. About 10% of the residents have moved to different types of accommodation after being discharged. This does not include moves that have taken place within the same type of accommodation.

Table 9.4 Residents placed in local authority establishments

---

1. *Catchment area*

Bexley	6 residents in mental handicap hostels
	1 resident in mental health hostel
Bromley	1 resident in mental handicap hostel
Greenwich	1 resident in mental handicap hostel
Kent	1 resident in mental handicap hostel
	1 resident in home for the elderly
Lambeth	2 residents in homes for the elderly
Lewisham	1 resident in mental health hostel
	3 residents in mental handicap hostel
Southwark	1 resident in mental handicap hostel
	2 residents in homes for the elderly
	1 resident in sheltered flat for the elderly

2. *Out of catchment area*

Tower Hamlets	1 resident in mental handicap hostel
Camden	3 residents in a home for the elderly
East Sussex	1 resident in hostel
Islington	1 resident in home for the elderly
Bedfordshire	1 resident in home for the elderly
Kensington and Chelsea	1 resident in home for the elderly

3. *Residents discharged from Grove Park Hospital placed in local authority establishments*

Bromley	8 residents in mental handicap hostel
	1 resident in home for the elderly
Lewisham	9 residents in mental handicap hostels
Greenwich	2 residents in hostels

New lives in the community

So far we have discussed what kinds of accommodation people are living in. Important as this is, it is still not as important as the opportunities that are presented to residents for acquiring new skills, experiencing new environments and activities, and generally learning how to become members of the community. Questionnaires were completed by care staff – and by a few residents themselves – for just under 100 residents, which dealt with the activities undertaken and the services used by these residents.

The aims in selecting these residents from all those discharged to the care of their districts were to ensure that residents of all degrees of handicap and residing in all types of accommodation were included in the survey. These

Table 9.5 Residents' moves after discharge

	Initial discharge							Placements, September 1988						
	Bexley	Bromley	Camberwell	Dartford/ Gravesham	Greenwich	Lewisham/ North Southwark	West Lambeth	Bexley	Bromley	Camberwell	Dartford/ Gravesham	Greenwich	Lewisham/ North Southwark	West Lambeth
Residential centre		51*	33	98			1	47*		40	72	′		1
NHS Hostel	21	69			68				34			53		
P/V	2	4	5	4		10	5	3	4	5	14		7	6
Staffed group homes	23	49	49	27		45	10	43	25	53	18	13	45	10
Independent homes						1	2		2		9	2	4	2
Family placement		1	1	1	2				1	1	8	2	1	
MIETS		2	1						2	1		1	1	
Other hospital		6	6		2	2	2		1		2	2	1	1
LA hostel	5					6		5		6		4	4	
Grove Park		1	1			15			11			13	13	
Misc.		2	2	1	2	1	2	1	1	2	1	2	1	1
Deaths											9	6	3	1
Interim training	1	15	15	1	44	2	4			5¹	1²	38³	4	4

* The residential centre accommodates 23 residents discharged from Grove Park Hospital.

1 No plans yet exist for these clients.
2 This client will move to a residential centre.
3 These clients will move to staffed group homes.

aims were only partially achieved. In selecting residents based on degrees of handicap, we relied on Wing's assessment of those residents who were in Darenth Park Hospital in August 1980, the baseline of her study. We relied on her assessments because they provided the only means of comparability across all seven districts, each district having chosen its own assessment method. The disadvantage of using these assessments was that they were eight years out of date by the time the hospital closed. As a result, we tended to have more people with mobility and general health problems than we had anticipated, due to the ageing of the population.

The second limitation was more significant. In order to get some impression of how the residents were coping in their new homes, a reasonable period of time needed to elapse between discharge and completion of the questionnaire, to allow them to settle and to have programmes of activities developed for them. The process and pace of discharge among the districts made it difficult to match up in advance residents and places of discharge. Further, as was mentioned (see Chapters 3 and 8), the programme of accommodation in several districts was so delayed that residents went into temporary accommodation. In several cases, it was those residents with quite severe handicaps and/or challenging behaviour who were among the last to be discharged, and the timing of our research did not allow for picking these up after a suitable interval in the community.

Our sample, therefore, cannot be said to be representative of the districts' new responsibilities for residents. We were not able to get agreement to include residents placed in private and voluntary accommodation. Nor were we able to look at the small number of residents who have individual placements in sheltered housing or Local Authority Part III homes. Our sample is therefore biased towards residents whose care has remained the responsibility of the NHS. Further, our information did not include any attempt to assess residents' skills or behaviour; this is the essence of Wing's study. However, it does represent the type of placements for all but 46 residents discharged post-1984.

We have shown (see Chapter 3) how the efforts of senior officers of South East Thames region to improve the conditions in which mentally handicapped people in the care of the health service reflected national concerns for this client group, and the policy objectives recommended. The 10 years of the Darenth Park project covered the period of time during which national policy changed from the *Better Services* model of care, which reserved a role, albeit much smaller, for hospital provision for the more severely handicapped or behaviourally disturbed residents, to a model of care based on the principle of normalization:

> Utilisation of means which are as culturally normative as possible, in order to establish and/or maintain personal behaviors and characteristics which are as culturally normative as possible. (Wolfensberger, 1972, p. 28)

This change had begun with the report of the Jay Committee (1979), was boosted by publication of *An Ordinary Life* (King's Fund Centre, 1980), and was finally blessed by the DHSS *Care in the Community* (1983b). Shortly after, it was accepted that almost all people with a mental handicap should live in the community; severity of handicap should not automatically be a deterrent.

Along with placing people with a mental handicap in ordinary housing, policy and practice began to spell out other aspects of service provision which quality services should consider: individual service plans; integrated health, social, education services; and support for establishing social networks.

It is the type of accommodation which has come to symbolize service models and most graphically reflects these policy changes. The three residential centres and purpose-built hostels represent the region's initial approach, agreed with the Darenth Park Steering Group in 1979, which followed the service recommendations of *Better Services* (DHSS, 1971) of no more than 200 new-build residential places on one site.

The change in policy objectives coincided with the 1982 restructuring of the NHS and new district staff quickly latched on to the implications of the new policy objectives for service provision. Between 1984 and 1989 approximately 300 places in group homes, the vast majority of which were in ordinary housing stock, were planned and developed. Plans for several hostels were cancelled, and one residential centre was scaled down in size to reduce the reliance on a form of residential provision no longer seen as desirable. The use of ordinary housing became the symbol of the new philosophy, in part because accommodation was the first and necessary step towards securing the presence of people with a mental handicap in the community in non-stigmatizing housing, and in part because it was the easiest aspect of normalization to fulfil.

At the same time, research and evaluative studies were beginning to demonstrate that it was possible to care for people even with a severe degree of mental handicap in the community in a way which was no less effective than hospital care, and in some respects more successful in that it stimulated a higher degree of skills, development and appropriate behaviour. Several small-scale studies showed that adaptive behaviour, IQ and skills development occurred to a greater degree in smaller, more normalized environments (Locker *et al.*, 1984; MacEachon, 1983; Conroy *et al.*, 1982; Witt, 1981; Thompson and Carey, 1980; Race and Race, 1979).

A major study in the UK was conducted in Wessex RHA, evaluating the changeover from total health service reliance on hospital care to the creation of 25-place community units and then smaller group homes in communities. The principal finding of the first phase of the study was that community units were feasible alternatives to hospital care, showing that gains in skills such as feeding, washing, dressing, appropriate social behaviour were greater among adults and children living in community units than in hospital (Smith *et al.*, 1980). Researchers went on to examine precisely the same issues for clients living in small group homes and again found higher levels of staff-client interaction, appropriate client behaviour and lower levels of inappropriate behaviour were achieved in small group homes than in larger community units or institutions (Thomas *et al.*, 1986) and higher levels of participation in activities (e.g. Saxby *et al.* 1986).

Many of the studies, however, admit that while community units or group homes seem to facilitate appropriate changes in clients, it is not clear how much should be attributed to size of unit and how much to other factors, such as staff training and support, commitment to philosophy of care, client mix and others. Bella (1976) reviewed various studies, concluding that care is generally more adequate in smaller units but small units also demonstrate considerable variation in standards of care, a conclusion reached by Pratt *et al.* (1980) as well. Changes in the environment do not seem to make much difference to clients' lives unless accompanied by other changes. Dalgleish (1983) examined some of the Sheffield Development project units and concluded that the physical environment had been improved in the newer units but that the actual management practices within the units had not changed very much so that the social environment still resembled that of large institutions. Tyerman and Spencer (1980) compared a new purpose-built ward and a superficially upgraded one and found in the new ward higher levels of positive activities and lower negative behaviour, such as inactivity, but little change in communication and interaction, and fewer self-care skills; they pointed to the need for more rigorous self-help training programmes.

A move to the community, in itself, seems to be least effective in providing means for clients to interact with non-handicapped people and develop social contacts and friendships away from the staff (Schalock and Lilley, 1986; Evans *et al.*, 1987).

Our observations of the different types of accommodation and the reports of clients' activities fit very well with the results of research discussed above. In general, greater efforts towards implementing ideas about normalization were found in group homes, or in units run as group homes, but some examples were found in all types of accommodation. It was also evident that homes in which staff had considerable experience of working with people with mental handicap, a greater commitment to normalize, and/or a more confident personality efforts at implementing services based on the principal of normalization were more consistent and seemed more successful. This, perhaps, does no more than reflect the immaturity of the infrastructure of services-training, management support systems, monitoring; the houses are in place but services still need developing. In completing the questionnaires, we could not help but make some observations about residents in their new homes and notice some of the differences among the types of accommodation. What follows is principally a descriptive account of the new units and the kinds of activities residents in them undertake.

Residential centres

There are three residential centres, although the one in Camberwell is considerably smaller than the other two (42 as opposed to 77 and 80 places).

Camberwell's residential centre is also managed by the Southwark Mental Handicap Consortium on behalf of a housing association, and this too makes it different from the other centres.

Each residential centre was built as a series of separate houses. Archery House, having been designed earliest, is the least like ordinary housing, having the largest units (four buildings of 20 places each). Its location is only marginally conducive towards the residents mixing in the community, because there are NHS buildings on two sides and the local council refuse dump in front. Each building at Archery House is divided into two wings: each wing has four single bedrooms and two bedrooms that sleep three each, and living and dining areas which also serve as pathways to the bedrooms. There is also a kitchen which is shared between the two wings. Breakfast is prepared by the unit staff, but the midday and evening meals are prepared centrally and sent in. Domestic staff are attached to each unit and there is a housekeeper who looks after the resident's clothes among other things. Sheets and towels are supplied from a central laundry. All units have been built to accommodate people in wheelchairs.

Bassetts Village consists of nine houses, each with their own front door and full range of facilities, including kitchen, living and dining rooms, staff office and a mixture of single and double bedrooms. All meals are prepared in the house and residents are encouraged to help with the shopping, cooking, washing up, and setting of the table. They are also encouraged to make their own tea and coffee and simply help or be in the kitchen when they want. There are no domestic staff, and the care team is expected to encourage the residents to help with the cleaning, especially their own rooms. The residents do get reward money for helping out in a variety of ways around the house. All of the laundry is done within the house. The houses are located in the midst of a residential area, but it is quite a walk to the nearest large shopping precinct and to local buses.

The third centre is designed as a series of self-contained bungalows, accommodating either six or eight residents each. They are equipped in a similar fashion to those at Bassetts Village, a mixture of single and double bedrooms. As at Bassetts Village, the staff are responsible for cleaning and cooking; each house has a housekeeper to help with these tasks. Bowley Close is located close to the shops and public transport, but they are an uphill walk away, making it difficult for some elderly residents to get out much.

Two of the three residential centres have a fairly domestic feel about them, and the care staff try to involve the residents in a range of domestic chores and encourage them to look after themselves and their own needs as much as possible. All three centres have a preponderance of elderly or wheelchair-bound residents, because of their need for ground floor accommodation. To some extent, this has tended to limit what is reasonable for the residents to undertake. Each centre also has at least one house of younger residents with more difficult behaviour problems.

Another feature shared by the centres is the lack of space provided by the purpose-built houses. Building to DHSS cost limits means that only about

80% of the recommended space allowances can be achieved because of the high level of construction costs in the south-east. Eight or nine residents take up a lot of room, and eight seating places plus a few side-tables and a TV take up the entire living room space. With one or more residents in wheelchairs, the living/dining rooms become crowded. Further, these homes were intended for eight residents, but this ignored that there would always be staff on duty – at least another three places at the dining table. The staff at each centre said they found the houses a bit cramped and thought the residents would benefit from more space and living with fewer people.

Not every house in each residential centre was visited, but among those that were, there were contrasting features. Two of the three centres were run as described above, much more on the lines of a domestic home than the third centre. The intention to make life as ordinary as possible was reflected in the importance attached to residents doing things for themselves or with staff, and getting off the campus as much as possible. This was dependent on several factors: the number of staff on duty and thus available to take people out singly or in pairs; the availability of transport for residents whose mobility was restricted; and the interests of the residents themselves.

The staffing levels did not differ greatly between the houses: each had two or three daytime staff (although one house had four). What did vary a lot were the number of residents staying at home during the day. In one centre, at least half the people in the home went to the day centre five days a week, and several others went two or three times a week for half days. In the second centre, most residents went to the day centre only two days a week, because the centre was not yet fully staffed. In the third centre, residents went over to the day centre for specific sessions which interested them: needlecraft, yoga, adult literacy, communication groups. One 72-year-old woman went to six classes a week – domestic skills, fitness for living, needlework, social club, music and movement, and art.

Besides going to the day centre, the residents had other ways of spending their time. Several went to church or synagogue regularly. Almost all went shopping, many several times a week. One person went horse-riding regularly. Others liked to potter about and do things around the home – washing up, making cups of tea for others, dusting and tidying their own rooms. One woman changed significantly after being given a hearing aid: the staff said she now asked for things, showed initiative by doing things off her own bat, and reminded staff if they had forgotten to do something for her.

The contrasting management styles of the residential centres reflect most of the issues raised in previous research: the importance of autonomy for the staff of the unit (King *et al.*, 1971); the size of the living unit rather than the overall size of the institution (Bella, 1976); increased levels of staff-client interaction in more normalized settings (Thomas *et al.*, 1986), to highlight just a few of the points. The residential centres demonstrate the significance of geographic location as either facilitating or hindering participation in the community or use of community facilities; the closer were shops and cafés, the more often residents got out to these, despite other difficulties.

Hostels

There were three purpose-built hostels, one of which took the form of three houses side-by-side so that in essence they functioned as group homes; the second consisted of two separate flats and one house, 24 places in total; the third consisted of four 8-place flats, two upstairs and two downstairs, and a communal social room and some offices on site as well. Another hostel was housed in a former convalescent unit for elderly people, handed over to the mental handicap services in 1981. Finally, there was a very large house, originally used by the Greenwich Hospital Management Committee, which had over the years become attached to Leybourne Grange Hospital. When the London Borough of Bromley was transferred from the catchment area of Leybourne Grange to Darenth Park in the early 1970s, this hostel went with Bromley where it was located. It was in a very small community and it was agreed with the local inhabitants that the hostel would be used for very mildly handicapped women only.

The purpose-built hostels had very different atmospheres. In one, the hostel was a home for life or until the resident wanted to move on, and the emphasis was on creating a domestic environment. Although each flat had its own complement of staff, interconnecting doors between the two downstairs and two upstairs flats were left unlocked and there were frequent comings and goings of staff from the flats, the staff officer on site and others which made the flat feel more like a hospital ward than a private home. Many of the residents were elderly, and wanted a quiet life. In the flat visited, residents were aged 42, 56, 67, 71, 73, 76, 79 and 80 years. Even the 80-year-old got out at least once a week to the local shops, as well as several times over a 6-month period to cafés and restaurants and on outings with other people from the flat. Those that were able to use public transport by themselves went to different shopping centres, to a local pop-in parlour, visited friends who lived elsewhere or went to sports events. Most people had 1 week's holiday in the past year. Some of the residents went to a local authority day centre, though rarely full-time. Some adult education classes – flower arrangement and needlecraft – were provided at different times of the week by an ILEA tutor in the social room, and this at least gave some stimulation to those who found it difficult to get around.

The other purpose-built hostel had a different mission. It was to prepare its first 24 residents for moving to more independent living arrangements in ordinary minimally staffed houses. At the time of the visit to the hostel, one group had already moved out and considerable visiting went on between the house and some residents of the hostel. Speaking with staff and looking through the staff diaries of daily activities, the impression gained was of considerable activity – travelling by public transport, going to sessions at the day centre, innumerable shopping trips (one gentleman liked to go out each morning for his newspaper to a small shop down the road), cooking, baking and help with all household chores, a lot of visiting among the flats and visits to former residents who had moved out to the house or independent flats. The staff also undertook a lot of individual work with residents, e.g. taking individuals shopping or for a meal. The residents were beginning to develop their own interests and several were quite capable of pursuing these themselves – horse riding, swimming, local Gateway clubs. Group outings were also arranged to Biggin Hill, the West End of London, the theatre or restaurants.

The staff were also involved in counselling residents. One woman had a temper and the care staff spent time talking to her, teaching her to recognize when she was getting angry and ways of dealing with it, and how her outbursts affected others in the flat and spoiled things for herself. The staff praised her when they could see that she was trying to control her anger. There was a period when she refused to take any medication and this affected her behaviour; however, the staff were able to persuade her of the importance of the medication.

In the long-established hostel, there was a mixture of women residents, some of whom had lived there for many years, having come from Leybourne Grange, and others who began moving in since 1983. After consultation with neighbours, the hostel began accepting male residents in 1987. Of the 20 residents discharged to the hostel, only 2 were in their 40s, and 6 in their 50s. The average age was 61.6 years, with the eldest being 83 years old. However, there were few mobility problems since there was very little ground floor accommodation and the upper storey of the house was on different levels. The hostel as a whole housed 31 residents, but the staff had tried to create a more intimate atmosphere by forming smaller groupings with their own sitting rooms and dining areas.

The residents went to the local shops fairly frequently, the district's day centre for particular classes, the local Gateway club and were taken to London to see the Christmas lights. They used local hairdressers and bought their own clothes in the local shops. The staffing ratio was fairly low (13.8 staff for 31 residents), but this reflected that this was a more able-bodied group. However, the residents were ageing, and thus they placed greater demands on the staff. Despite the low staffing levels, the staff were able to take most residents out on their own once every week or so, usually a trip to a local shopping centre, to browse in the shops, to pick up knitting wool, to get a haircut or have a meal out. The limited availability of transport also constrained the staff's ability to take the residents out more.

One of the greatest assets that the hostel had was several acres of land, including an orchard and the remains of the kitchen garden, including derelict greenhouses. Some horticultural work involving the residents had already begun, but there were plans to expand this which involved bringing in other people to work with the residents.

Group homes

The group homes catered for between two and eight residents. The majority made use of existing housing stock and accommodated between three and five residents. It was apparent that many of these houses had a higher staff to resident ratio (2 : 1 was not unusual), especially those catering for residents with challenging behaviour (3 : 1, and 5 : 1 in one case). At the other end of the spectrum, in the houses that catered for the more able a ratio of 7 : 5 was not uncommon, and in one case it was 5 : 7.

It took the residents time to get used to living in much smaller houses compared to the Darenth Park wards. Some began by spending practically no time in their own bedrooms, and others by hardly coming out of their bedrooms. After a few months, most began to find a balance and appreciate their private space.

Almost all of the residents were involved in household chores, although those with very severe handicaps were able to do less; however, the staff were able to help even these residents – press the button to heat up a kettle, fill a kettle, put a tea bag in a cup, pour milk, or take plates from the table to the sink. In some cases, it looked a bit like tokenism. The resident was really paying no attention to what they were being asked to do, and even if guided in certain activities, they gave no recognition that they were performing that action.

When asked what more could be provided, staff suggested more organized day activities and social opportunities for making friends, so that residents could get out. A number of clients went to adult training centres once or twice a week. Others structured their week: collect money from the post office (Monday afternoon); swimming (Tuesday morning); wash clothes (Wednesday morning); tidy room (Wednesday afternoon); shop for food (Friday morning); church (Sunday). Some homes organized the staff and activities so that once a week each resident had a day with one staff member to him/herself. Others found new activities, such as watching horse racing on television and going to the races, or attending classes at a local adult education institute (AEI), e.g. gardening, cooking, music, woodwork, adult literacy, or computer classes. Houses often organized their own outings, either for an individual with special interests or for all of the residents together – this might be as simple as a walk in the park or hiring a mini bus to the coast. Some residents enjoyed a bus ride and part of their week's activity was to take a long bus ride. In general, staff made every effort to ensure that residents got out of the house once a day, if only to a local shop.

The activities which the residents got involved in may not seem very elaborate or perhaps exciting, but they represent a change from life in Darenth Park. Here are some examples:

- One resident gets up, chooses his own clothes and dresses himself (this he did not do when at Darenth Park); gets his own breakfast; goes to the shops; helps with the sweeping and hoovering; listens to music in his room.
- A resident goes to a cook-and-eat class once a week, and also does yoga and pottery at an AEI. She does a lot of work around the house – cooking, washing up, laundry, making her bed and shopping. She enjoys going to pubs and a café with friends. As she is deaf, she is now learning Maketon.

- A 74-years-old man who is confined to a wheelchair begins his day by getting up between 7.30 and 8.00. He runs his own bath, washes and dresses himself and makes his breakfast around 9.00. He then spends some time in his room tidying things. He likes to go to the post office to get his benefits and manages to go out every day. He has a specially adapted cooker and he chooses his meals from menu cards with pictures. He enjoys listening to music, watching football and going out for meals.

This fairly rosy picture needs to be balanced by pointing out that there were some residents who were not happy living in the community, and whom the staff found difficult to motivate. It was evident from one or two of the homes visited, that some staff were uncertain of what to try out with the residents – the staff tended to feel uneasy if residents were just sitting in front of the television but they could offer no alternatives.

What also was conveyed during the visit was the considerable pride many staff felt in the accomplishments of their residents since living in their new homes. Many of their accomplishments may seem quite small – choosing what to wear, what to eat, when to go out, what to do outside – but they represent a very different lifestyle from that they had been used to in Darenth Park. For many, though, it was several months before they felt able to express their own views – 'you're the nurse, you know what I want' was the way one man responded when asked whether he wanted tea or coffee.

In brief

The brief impressions gained through collecting information for the costing exercise have begun to show that some accommodation facilities change in residents by location, by a domestic atmosphere which helps to create a different set of relationships between staff and residents, and by intimacy of contact brought about by smaller numbers. All accommodation was of a much higher standard than the hospital, following more closely traditional domestic arrangements which afford some degree of privacy (although the majority of residents in hostels and residential centres share a bedroom, something unlikely to occur in currently planned facilities). All residents for whom information was collected have seemed to gain in other aspects as well: respect shown to them by the staff, a greater awareness by staff of the right of residents to be involved in deciding what happens to them, in choice, and of the desirability of getting out into the community as much as possible, despite difficulties.

Despite the differences in the main types of accommodation, residents from all three types of settings have moved on to the more independent living arrangements. With these points in mind, it is reasonable to say that some degree of 'normalization' has been achieved for all residents, even if limited. What would be needed for residents to reach their potential and to lead as varied a life as possible would be further development of staff training, support and supervision; individual programme plans for each resident; a method of monitoring, evaluating and acting upon their evaluation. None of the Darenth Park residents were yet living in such a service system.

CHAPTER 10

The cost of reprovision

The wider economic literature

Despite the fact that financial considerations have been so important in affecting politicians' attitudes to deinstitutionalization, it is surprising how little hard economic evidence there is. What does exist is largely confined to the field of mental illness, not mental handicap, and much of the work has been done in other countries. Very few studies in either case take account of the full range of economic costs and even fewer portray the impact of complete hospital closure. The most frequent approach has been to take a matched sample of long stay residents or patients and those being cared for by community placements and organizations. Often the result has been to underestimate the costs of community care either because the studies exclude the full range of social costs or because they understate the eventual cost of moving out the most handicapped. This tendency is eliminated if we study the outcome of complete closure. No other complete closure has been costed in the UK and very few in the international literature. This is the significance of the Darenth Park study.

Cost benefit studies of non hospital care strategies for the mentally ill were pioneered in the United States in the 1970s (Sheenan and Atkinson, 1974; Cassell *et al.*, 1972; Endicott *et al.*, 1978). The most comprehensive was the study by Weisbrod *et al.* (1980). There were two studies in Canada and Australia (Fenton *et al.*, 1982; Hoult *et al.*, 1983). More recently Knapp and colleagues at Kent University have been concerned with estimating the effects of closing Friern Barnet, a large London mental hospital (Knapp *et al.*, 1987).

Most of the studies of the mentally ill suggest that community care can be cheaper but the results are more ambiguous than is sometimes suggested. For example, the very careful influential study by Weisbrod *et al.* (1980) suggested that the treatment costs of the experimental community programme were more than that of institutional care. The positive result that the programme produced was the result of enhanced benefits to patients and the community which were given monetary values. The most important, by far, was the higher earnings that individuals were able to sustain in the community.

The more recent work by Knapp and Beecham (1989) in Britain does suggest that community care can be a less costly option even when the whole range of alternative economic costs are taken into account. Again it is important to stress this does not reflect evidence from a full closure.

Work on mental handicap has been much more sparse and the results somewhat different. In the first place care of the mentally handicapped is usually continuous rather than intermittent. Especially in the case of the moderately and profoundly handicapped it means close and interactive personal care. In a large institution there are certain economies of scale, for example during the night. In a very small group home this is less possible. Secondly, only in very few cases is there full or even sheltered participation in the labour force. Thus monetary benefits are difficult to achieve and certainly have not been reflected in the literature. The only comparable study outside the United Kingdom which we have been able to find was undertaken to evaluate the court ordered closure of Pennhurst Center which served the South East Region of Pennsylvania and housed 1154 people in 1978 (Conroy and Bradley, 1985). In many ways the comparison with Darenth is close and the differences intriguing. The pressure for closure came not through political action but through law suits brought on behalf of two residents claiming the constitution gave individuals the right to be cared for in the least restrictive setting. The Judge ordered that suitable alternative community services be provided for all the residents and for similar individuals. Later orders required that individual personal plans had to be submitted to the court specifying alternative care. All children had to be out of the institution by September 1979 and the Center closed by September 1986 at the latest. An evaluation of the whole process was undertaken and a research report published covering the first five years progress (Conroy and Bradley, 1985). Research is continuing.

The follow up of a sample of 176 people showed that while those living in the centre from 1978 to 1980 showed little change in adaptive behaviour scores or their independent living capacity, when moved to community settings their scores improved sharply, beginning to level out again three or four years later. 'The adaptive behaviour growth displayed by people who moved to (community placements) under the court order is literally ten times greater than the growth displayed by matched people who are still at Pennhurst' (p. 315). Residents expressed mixed views about leaving, but were happier once they had moved.

The cost analysis is interesting for the investigators not only tried to compare the costs of the original Center, or hospital, with the new smaller scale community services but also tried to explain the differences. The average annual cost at the Pennhurst Center was $45,000 a year in 1981/2. This was higher than the US national average cost of $34,000, and higher than the UK equivalent, by any measure, as we shall see.

The cost analysis of new forms of care was on a slightly different basis to that in the Darenth study. The evaluators took a sample of residential care facilities and took their average costs. They also took the average costs of facilities used by residents like day care centres. They did not, as we did, and as Knapp has done, follow up use of services on an individual basis. This reduces the variance in per capita figures. We know nothing about how much different residents used the facilities outside the residential centres. The costs of the small community living centres at $33,237 were less than living costs at the Pennhurst Center. The day care programmes were slightly less expensive and the medical costs a lot less.

The evaluators were, however, cautious about the long term. The variation in costs was very wide. The main reason for the lower costs in residential settings was lower staff costs. This in turn was the result of paying lower wages. Most staff were 'second earners' (that is to say women!) in newly established and non-unionized facilities. They suggest, sensibly, that these costs differences are likely to narrow as such facilities become the norm. It is interesting that precisely the opposite salary differential has been true in Britain. Local authority social work pay scales have been higher than those of nursing staff. Again, the higher medical costs at Pennhurst derived from the peculiarities of the funding of American Medicaid which encouraged high billing for hospital procedures.

In short, the cost advantages in the Pennhurst case may owe more to the peculiarities of American health care economics and be short term in their effect.

The one piece of early British evidence, from York (Wright and Haycox, 1985), on the relative costs of small scale facilities for the mentally handicapped compared to a long stay hospital suggested that such facilities were more expensive.

Knapp and Beecham (1989) have evaluated the economic cost differences between long stay institutions and demonstration projects to which people moved. Their preliminary results cover the mentally ill, the mentally handicapped, the physically disabled and the elderly. Most of the mentally handicapped, however, moved to staffed group homes. Their calculation of the whole range of service costs using the same methodology as ours suggested an average cost which was slightly lower in the group homes compared to the hospital. In neither the Wright and Haycox nor in the Knapp and Beecham case was the comparison between closure and complete reprovision. To the best of our knowledge these are the first results from such an analysis.

Having reviewed the limited comparable previous cost studies we can explain our own approach.

Methodology

As explained in the previous chapter a sample of residents moving out of Darenth Park was chosen to include examples of people in the whole range of alternative facilities and those suffering from different levels of disability. We aimed at a sample of 100. In the end, we obtained details of 93 residents now in alternative facilities. We considered it important to base the costings on the experience of individuals rather than broad averages. Many previous studies underestimated the diversity of people's needs. Thus, we interviewed residents as well as care managers or their equivalent, to find out what visits residents made to what kind of facility and what actual social security benefits they were drawing. (Care staff were not always well informed about the benefits. They often got the total right but were confused about the nature of the benefit.) Our methodology closely follows that of Knapp *et al.* (1987), though we adapted the same interview schedule for mentally handicapped residents. Our study uses the same methodology as Sheill and Wright (1988) and the DHSS (1987) option appraisal approach. Our own study has its limitations, however. The measures of disability are those assigned to residents by Lorna Wing, in her parallel study begun in 1980. Older residents, in particular, would have deteriorated between then and the time they were moved – between 1980 and August 1988. Nevertheless, some common measurement point was necessary. Reassessment at the point of transfer would have been ideal but was not available. We were unable to interview care staff in any of the private or voluntary facilities despite attempts to do so.

Unfortunately, we possess outcome measures for only some of the residents. For those who moved in the early 1980s, Lorna Wing's study gives us an unparalleled set of information. The results are reported in detail in her interim reports (Wing, 1984, 1989). They relate mainly to the residents who moved into the small hospital and the larger units and not into the group homes and small units opened later. Overall, her test scores show relatively little change in the residents living in the new facilities. Our observations of the smaller, more informal settings suggest that they have produced more changes in social behaviour and more contentment. This is a purely subjective view and must remain as such until Wing's follow-up study is published. We are therefore comparing, at the most pessimistic, care outcomes that are no worse than in Darenth Park, and facilities which providers and relatives (see Wing, 1989) consider to have improved. What then are the comparable costs?

The distinction between costs and finance

We have to distinguish at the outset between the economic cost of the alternative kinds of provision from the question of 'who pays?' The economic cost is a measure of the resources used to provide care for the resident – the recurrent cost of staff, building maintenance, food, medical care, transport, and the capital cost of the buildings and sites involved. The financial complications concern who pays for this – the DHSS, the NHS, or a local authority. We therefore conducted the analysis in two parts. We first calculated for each individual the scale of resources used in his or her care and

Table 10.1 The economic costs of reprovision

Resource	Valuation method	Price basis
A. *Capital*		
Land	market value (housing)	1987
Buildings	construction costs (assume 60-year life, 5% discount rate)	1987
B. *Running costs*		
Staff	gross salaries employment costs	1987–8 accounts
Non-staff	other current expenditure	
C. *Agency services*		
Medical		
Dental	costs per consultation length estimated	PSSRU estimates (1987–8 prices), costs per minute
Paramedical		
Day care	costs per attendance	day centre accounts (1987–8 prices)
D. *Community services*		
Education costs	costs per class attended	as for 1987–8
Bus passes	at cost	
Other services	assume minimal marginal cost	
E. *Personal consumption*		
	DHSS personal allowance, mobility allowance or other	as in 1987–8

Note: Sum of A − E = annual economic cost per place.

then who paid for it. In practice, we were not faced with calculating the cost of family care because not one of our sample returned to live with his or her family. In the group as a whole, only 24 of 1138 people who moved after 1978 returned to live with their families or relations, and only 6 did so in the period we were studying in depth. We were unable to obtain access to their details and any sample would not have been representative.

There is one case where a slight blurring of the conceptual distinction between provision and finance occurs, and that is with private consumption. We should, in theory at least, include an estimate of all personal consumption over and above food that is provided by the hostel or group home, e.g. money for cigarettes, outings, snacks, etc. In practice, most people only have their personal allowance from the DHSS; some may have a private income, but we have only taken into account the public contribution to consumption financed by the DHSS.

The broad types of cost we were seeking to calculate are set out in Table 10.1 and the possible sources of funds are set out in Table 10.2. Both tables are taken from Sheill and Wright (1988) and formed the conceptual basis of our analysis.

Table 10.2 Who pays? The possible distribution of financial costs

Funding Agency – budget	Types of residential provision					
	NHS hospital	NHS group home	Local hostel	Authority group home	Private or voluntary	
					Nursing	Group home
1. National Health Service						
Health and community service	√	√	—	—	—	—
Family practitioner committee	—	√	√	√	√	√
2. Local authority social services department						
Residential	—	—	√	√	—	—
Day	—	√	√	√	√	√
Domiciliary	—	√	√	√	√	√
3. Department of Health and Social Security[a]						
Income support	—	—	√	√	√	√
Board and lodgings	—	—	—	—	√	√
Housing benefit	—	√	—	√	—	√
SDA/mob allowance	√	√	√	√	√	√
Attendance allowance	—	—	—	—	—	√
4. Department of the Environment						
Housing Association grants	—	—	—	—	—	√
Hostel deficit grants	—	—	—	—	—	√
5. Others						
MSC	√	√	√	√	√	√
Informal	√	√	√	√	√	√
Others	√	√	√	√	√	√

[a] Entitlement to some social security benefits is dependent on the discretion of local social security officers, and their judgement about the type of facility in which a mentally handicapped person resides.

Source: Sheill and Wright (1988).

Costing reprovision

Our first task was to calculate the capital cost of the new facilities in which the residents were housed. This involved expressing the original cost of construction in 1987–8 prices and producing an annuity cost, i.e. the annual cost of the capital resources used up per resident. Following Treasury and DHSS (1987) guidelines (discussed by Knapp *et al.*, 1987, and Shiell and Wright, 1988), we assumed a 60-year life for the buildings and a discount rate of 5%. We also estimated the site value of NHS development. We assumed a rather lower than average Greater London-wide price per hectare for housing land and that only 50% of any site area could be used for housing. In combination, this gives us the annual capital cost for each facility. Dividing by the number of residents in the facility gives us the average capital cost per resident in each facility.

Table 10.3 An individual cost schedule for community residents

---

Types of service

---

1. NHS hospital
     in-patient
     out-patient

2. NHS hostel or residential centre

3. NHS – FPC
     GP surgery
     home visit
     dentist
     chiropodist
     physiotherapist
     psychologist
     psychiatric service
     speech therapy
     day centre
     medication

4. Local authority services
     day centre
     hostel
     bus pass
     education classes

5. Housing Association group home
     current expenditure

6. DHSS benefits
     mobility, etc.
     personal

The next step was to calculate the running cost of the facility in which each of the residents in our sample was living. This was usually quite straight-forward. Separate accounts existed for each NHS facility and, though this was more difficult to extract, for each group home as well. We needed to find out what the staff costs were, whether they were met by the NHS, hostel deficit grant or local authority, and the running expenses. From this, an average running cost per resident was obtained. Accounts were available for 1987–8 in most cases. In one case, spending for 1988–9 was revalued to 1987–8 prices, and November 1986 prices were revalued upwards.

Finally, it was necessary to fill in a questionnaire for each resident which detailed what external health services they had used and for how long. We adapted the PSSRU questionnaire devised by Knapp and his colleagues in their study of the reprovision of Friern Barnet. The facilities used by the mentally handicapped were slightly different. The headings we used are given in Table 10.3. Knapp's costings were adopted and amended to 1987–8 prices. DHSS benefits were added.

The cost of hospital care

The true relative cost of reprovision can only be determined when we know what it would have cost *not* to reprovide the hospital. The option to do nothing at all had become politically unviable as we saw in the earlier chapters. Just what it would have cost to keep Darenth Park going as a hospital is very difficult to estimate and depends on a range of assumptions. Economics at this point becomes an inexact science. The best we can do, and it is a lot better than doing nothing, is to give a range of estimates. It is important to make some sort of estimates in case people view the costs of reprovision with some anxiety, forgetting that it would also have been costly to rebuild a 2000-bed Victorian hospital! No one was proposing to rebuild Darenth Park, of course, but the Region's previous policy dated from the government's Hospital Plan of 1962, which planned to 'upgrade' the buildings. The minutes of a Hospital Board meeting in 1973 put the cost at between £2 million and £5 million. Assuming that the costs would have overrun if the plan had ever been implemented, it is reasonable to take £5 million at 1973 prices as a modest estimate. Even so, this would have been only a temporary measure. In 1970, there were about 1500 residents in Darenth Park. At the same time, the Region was planning to provide more accommodation off site for about 400–450 residents at a capital cost of £3.5 million. Archery House was an early design and gives us perhaps a more realistic measure of the costs rebuilding on the site would have involved. These alternative capital costs have to be expressed in 1987–8 prices, and the costs annualized assuming a 60-year life of the asset and a discount rate of 5% – the same assumptions as we used for the new capital facilities in the community.

There was also an 'opportunity cost' involved, i.e. the inability to sell the site or use it for other purposes. To calculate this we need to know how much it would sell for in the open market. The value of the 200-acre site would depend, essentially, on what the planning authorities, and ultimately the Secretary of State for the Environment, would permit the site to be used for. Darenth Park is in London's Green Belt and guidance about the Department's policy on granting permission for alternative use of such sites was set out by the Department of the Environment in 1987 (Circular 12/87). Where feasible, the Circular states, existing buildings should be used for other purposes. Where this is not possible, a site can be redeveloped, but no more densely than at present, and at no greater height. A similar case had arisen at Shenfield Hospital. At the time of writing, the outcome of negotiations about Darenth Park's site was not clear. The margins of valuation were therefore very wide. As agricultural land the site may be worth only £100 000. If developed for housing, however, the site could be worth £50 million or more. We have assumed alternative site values.

What was it costing to keep residents in Darenth Park in terms of running expenses? It is again by no means clear precisely what to base this calculation on. The average costs in 1970 are misleading because there was already

Table 10.4 The average annual costs (1987 prices) of hospital care at Darenth Park

Average recurrent expenditure per resident	
NHS costs (1981 standards and number of resident)	12 490
Local authority social work input	52
Total	12 542
Annual capital cost	
A. Construction	
(a) cost of 'upgrading' in 1973	660
(b) cost of new provision per place in 1973	3123
(c) Archery House equivalent including day centre	2750
B. Site cost	
(a) redevelopment low density for housing	880
(b) redevelopment higher density	1760
Personal consumption expenditure (DHSS funded)	429
Total Cost	
Median assumption	≃16 600
Top assumption	≃19 000

strong ministerial pressure to improve standards and this was accepted by the Region. It seemed more appropriate to take the recurrent costs in 1982 when our sample of residents were all still accommodated in Darenth Park. These too must be calculated in 1987–8 prices. Our best estimate is an annual average of about £12 500 for all residents. This average will have varied according to the extent of handicap, but we have no means of knowing how much extra resources a severely handicapped person received in hospital at the time. To NHS average costs we must add the social work contribution paid for by the local authorities – a very small sum – and the social security payments secured by residents.

We are now in a position to present a rough range of costs for keeping the hospital as it was (see Table 10.4). All costs are expressed in 1987–8 prices. The total annual economic cost of replacing Darenth Park on its own site could have been £16 100 per resident, though possibly closer to £19 000.

Costs of reprovision

New services vary with the degree of incapacity suffered by the residents. We were fortunate to be able to use the assessments undertaken by Dr Wing in 1980 (for a detailed explanation of the instruments used, see Wing, 1989). We grouped the sample residents into four groups:

Table 10.5 The average annual recurrent costs (£) of reprovision (1987–8 prices)

	Recurrent[a]	Personal consumption[b]	Total
NHS hostel (traditional style)	14 780		15 495
NHS residential centres (group home style)	19 000	715	19 715
All NHS hostels and residential centres	16 066		16 781
Group homes	24 808	757	25 523
Including average annual costs of:			
Hospital care			
in-patient			370
out-patient attendances			26
Family practitioner, community health service, day centre, medication			424
Local authority services			594

[a] Including use of NHS hospital care and community services, GPs, etc.
[b] DHSS-financed only.

1 Socially impaired with behaviour problems.
2 Socially impaired but amenable.
3 Sociable with behaviour problems.
4 Sociable and amenable.

A separate analysis by age would have been misleading. As we have already seen, the level of handicap increased in the younger age group, because of changing admissions policies.

Recurrent costs of reprovision

Table 10.5 shows the average recurrent costs of reprovision in the different kinds of accommodation. The lowest recurrent costs are to be found in the larger, more institutional NHS hostels where average staffing and running costs were just over £11 000, plus day centre costs for some residents of £2000. The mean cost was about £14 780. This included a limited use of NHS community services, or the GP and dentist. Costs of other NHS facilities, which were much more like group homes, were more expensive – just over £19 000.

The resource costs of the more intensively staffed group homes were higher still, though the total was met out of several different budgets. The NHS usually paid for some of the staff in these homes. According to the severity of handicap, staff costs varied from £10 000 to £50 000 in one case. The median staffing costs were £16 000, but could be as much as £20 000. The other costs involved in running a house plus administrative overheads varied from about

Table 10.6 The range of average recurrent costs per resident per annum (excluding personal consumption)

	£10 000–14 999	£15 000–19 999	£20 000–24 999	£25 000–29 999	£30 000–39 999	£40 000–49 999	£50 000+	All residents in sample
No. of residents	19	31	27	5	7	3	1	93

£3000 a year to £8500 or more in a few cases. The overall mean recurrent cost of group homes, excluding DHSS payments for personal spending, was £24 808 (1987–8 prices). Again these figures include the use of local services.

The costs of day centre provision varied and are included in the above figures. Some residents only used these facilities on two or three days a week, others on five days. NHS day centre costs were lower than local authority costs, averaging about £1600 per person. Local authority provision was often double this figure, and in one case was £6000 p.a. The costs of out-patient and in-patient care were significant for a few individuals, but averaged out at about £400 p.a. The wide range of average costs per resident is shown in Table 10.6.

Table 10.7 shows how the average recurrent costs varied between types of handicap. These are less important than the type of facilities. Overall, the average recurrent costs in the newer facilities and group homes were higher than for Darneth Park. Given the reasons behind the closure of Darenth Park in the first place, and the efforts to find good quality alternative care on an individualized basis, this is not surprising – good 'community care' does not come cheap. Those residents who were transferred from Darenth Park early on to private homes or board and lodgings were not included in our sample. To take account of this, we have produced a weighted average figure for the cost of all placements as at September 1988 (see Table 10.9). This gives an average recurrent cost, excluding personal consumption, of £20 715. The likely reason for these relatively high costs compared to other studies lies, we believe, in the fact that the most handicapped proved very expensive to provide for and that they were the last to leave Darenth Park, something the earlier studies may have underestimated.

Table 10.7 Average recurrent costs (£) by type of resident (excluding DHSS personal payments, 1987–8 prices)

	NHS facilities	Group homes	All
Socially impaired with behaviour problems	16 867	27 760	24 755
Socially impaired but amenable	13 794	21 147	18 635
Sociable with behaviour problems	15 701	28 554	23 412
Sociable and amenable	18 128	26 479	22 095

Table 10.8 Average annual capital costs (£) of
reprovision, 1987–8 (including sites)

NHS hostels	3500
Group homes	4271

Capital costs of reprovision

The annualized capital costs of new facilities should be treated with caution.
The facilities were built at different times and an average price adjustment is
only a rough guide to 1987–8 prices. Site costs were difficult to estimate
where the sites were already in NHS hands and part of a wider NHS complex.
In these cases, we used average Greater London prices per hectare as a rough
guide but took a rather lower figure since the sites were not ideal. All in all, the
capital figures are no more than a rough order of magnitude to make the
reader aware that such costs are present and in London can be considerable. It
is inherent in reprovision in a large urban centre that this will be the case. The
results are given in Table 10.8.

The overall costs

We present our estimates of the overall average costs of reprovision in Table
10.9.

Table 10.9 Average annual total costs (£) of reprovision, 1987–8

	Recurrent	Personal consumption	Capital	Total
NHS hostels and centres	16 066	715	3500	20 281
Group homes	24 808	757	4271	29 836
Total weighted average	20 715	740	3800	25 255

Who has paid?

Having looked at the overall economic cost of reprovision, we need to know
who paid. Where the facility used by our sample is owned and run by the
NHS, then the NHS have funded it. Where the service is provided by a local
authority, we count it as being funded by the local authority unless they
received funding from the NHS. It is true, of course, that about half of this

Table 10.10 Financing reprovision costs (£) per annum, 1987–8

	NHS facilities		Group homes	
	£	%	£	%
Recurrent costs met by				
NHS hospitals, FPC and community	884	(5.5)	769	(3.1)
NHS care costs	14 665	(91.3)	15 310	(61.7)
Local authority	517	(3.2)	655	(2.6)
DSS	—		6669	(26.9)
DoE	—		1405	(5.7)
Totals	16 066	(100)	24 808	(100)

expenditure will have been met from central government grants. The more complex analysis involves group homes run by housing associations or where charges are levied on the resident and reimbursed on his or her behalf by the DSS. Housing associations not only charge rent, they also receive a capital subsidy from central government to reduce the revenue costs to a level that used to be equivalent to a 'fair rent' which could be paid out of housing benefit. We have not attempted to estimate this, but have calculated the portion of recurrent costs met by the hostel deficit grant. Here the source of the subsidy is the Department of the Environment via the Housing Corporation. The individual analysis of the sample residents enabled us to estimate how the funding for recurrent expenditure was divided between different governmental departments for each of the alternative kinds of provision (see Table 10.10).

It is evident that the social security budget made a considerable contribution (27%) to the financing of the move to group homes and the maintenance of residents. The Department of the Environment met 5.7%. This is only reasonable if the aim is for residents to lead more normal lives. The reduction in social security board and lodging benefits promised by the government could have a significant effect on the viable funding of hospital closure. Local authorities contributed very little in financial terms, between 2 and 3% of the cost.

In brief

There were wide variations in the annual cost of facilities. Small group homes which received funding from a variety of public sources had higher costs than the more institutionalized forms of residential care. Essentially, it seems the NHS had held its own contribution down but had relied on other sources to enhance the level of provision.

Overall, the recurrent annual costs of reprovision were subsequently more than care in the old large Victorian hospital that had been difficult to staff. That should really not come as a surprise. More humane care costs more.

Net capital costs depend so much on imponderables such as alternative use values and site acquisition that precise conclusions are unwise but the costs do not appear that different to reprovision on the old site.

CHAPTER 11

A *review: pointers for other closures*

At the outset we asked whether the British experience of psychiatric hospital closures mirror that in the United States. We have drawn a distinction between the problems posed by provision for the mentally ill in the community and the reprovision of services for the mentally handicapped. Long-term alternative facilities are easier to plan in the case of the latter. Darenth Park is but one case study. Nevertheless, as far as this case is concerned, the answer to our question is no: the worst US experience has not been mirrored, but more of the best has been. Throughout, Regional Health Authority officers strove to ensure that adequate alternative provision was made for all ex-residents of Darenth Park. Early on, their concern was, if anything, too protective. As we have seen, attempts at ensuring a common standard of facilities in every district failed. Individual districts wanted different things. The difficulties of obtaining sites and adequate finance helped to create a climate much more receptive to principles of normalization, and ordinary housing. The fact that such provision could mobilize money from sources other than the NHS was an important factor.

Regional leadership

When we submitted our interim report in1984 we had private doubts about whether the hospital would close at all. What the project illustrates first, then, is that public bureaucracies, for that is what the NHS is, *can* adapt and *can* learn from their mistakes, if they are well led. What emerged after 1983 was a new pattern of strong regional leadership with professional and technical support for those undertaking the reprovision locally, but with a maximum amount of financial devolution and minimal detailed capital control. That approach conforms well to the pattern of management exercised in some of the most successful large corporations, if we are to believe Peters and Waterman (1982), a 'tight–loose' relationship between the centre and the district and unit level managers. A number of important principles emerge:

1 *Continuing pressure to succeed.* The Darenth Park Project was initiated by regional officers and brought to conclusion by them. It was they who kept up the pressure when districts wanted more time, more money, more space. Understandable though these requests were, delay proved very deleterious to conditions in the hospital and the Region had to keep districts to a tight timetable as far as possible.

2 *Continuity.* During a time when local units were being reorganized several times and local officers came and went, the continuity of key officers within the Region was critical. The Chair of the Steering Group, Dame Audrey Emerton, remained a powerful force until the end. The appointment of a co-ordinator responsible for solving problems as they arose and a team of officers (the Task Force) who met regularly to further the project, was again important, as can be seen from a detailed record of events before and after 1983.

3 *Facilitating and 'empowering' change.* The funding policy enabled the Region to simplify what had been a complicated set of negotiations with each district about the mix of disabilities its residents had. By simplifying the funding arrangements, the regional treasurer let the districts know exactly how much money they could expect to receive for each resident. Moreover, it was possible for them to use that money to negotiate with other bodies like housing associations. Several officers frustrated by the internal works and design facilities were able to achieve results more quickly using external agencies.

4 *Incentives for action.* The funding policy gave the right incentives for action. It illustrates that it is not sufficient to rely on goodwill or bureaucratic altruism to achieve a policy goal. Appropriate financial incentives within public agencies are of critical importance.

5 *A shared philosophy.* Most participants came, eventually, to share a common philosophy of normalization or ordinary living. We shall see later that this still has unresolved problems, but it helped build a better understanding between social services departments and NHS officers.

6 *New styles of working.* The new approach had several distinct aspects. For clients, it represented an attempt to implement a model of care approximating to 'ordinary life' – to get away from those aspects of accommodation which were seen as depersonalizing and stigmatizing. For the districts, it represented a new freedom to negotiate locally the kinds of service provision they saw as desirable, in keeping with local tastes and preferences. For the Region, it represented a significant change in planning relationships, both with districts and with housing associations.

7 *Professional support.* By appointing a regional staff training co-ordinator, the Region was able to offer practical assistance and reassurance to those embarking on a new form of care and provision. By funding a back-up team that helped with the most disturbed residents, the districts were able to accept people they might have otherwise rejected.

8 *A brokerage role.* The districts' interests often differed and yet

agreements had to be made. In many instances, regional officers found themselves taking on a brokerage role, negotiating on behalf of, or easing the path towards negotiation by, the districts. It was often only at the regional level that issues unresolved by two districts could be sorted out. There was a need for someone to be seen to have the authority to make agreements and to have the means of making them stick. That was a role only the Region could fulfil.

9 *The headmaster (mistress) role.* When some districts or units fell behind, a tough reminder of responsibilities was, on occasion, necessary. The accountability reviews helped in this process.

10 *Tasks remain.* Despite the success achieved with the closure of Darenth Park and provision of alternative accommodation, two problems remain. First, some of the early schemes are, in modern terms, highly institutional. The patterns of daily activity and residents' behaviour has changed relatively little (Wing, forthcoming). There is still a need to evaluate and rethink some of the facilities. Secondly, several outstanding problems have to be faced concerning the new style group homes. They have been created, but how can they be sustained and evaluated? Many are isolated and employ young, inexperienced staff. How can the quality of care be sustained?

Districts' response

The districts, too, have gained some useful experience in the management of change, in addition to learning to work with the Region:

1 *Involvement from the beginning.* Recognizing that other agencies and individuals have valuable contributions to make to service provision and to the acceptance of people with a learning disability, it makes sense to include them from the outset so that they exert real influence rather than a token consultation.

2 *Core of staff.* Districts developing new services need to employ a senior core of staff to plan and oversee the implementation of the services before they begin to fulfil the management functions which will be their long-term responsibilities. It is very easy to underestimate the range of decisions that need to be made when developing new services and how early ill-conceived decisions create problems for the future.

3 *The range of services.* Though housing is of prime importance, officers must be aware of the much wider range of services needed by people with learning disabilities. Serious efforts need to be made to educate people as to what is available locally and to train staff in providing for those with disabilities. In particular, more attention needs to be paid to what people with learning disabilities want – social activities, work, to be close to friends.

4 *The high costs of creating a service.* Because senior staff are needed from the outset and because it may take up to two or more years to develop a service before receiving clients, districts need to be prepared to spend money on development work. Doing it on the cheap results in a cheap service.

5 *Importance of allies.* In several districts, many services were not understood by DHA members and thus they did not defend them. They needed to be persuaded that the new services were a legitimate part of the NHS.

6 *Staffing needs.* Districts need to make a special effort when recruiting staff so as to balance their age and experience. Drawing on a wider range of people who have something more to offer services, requires more than just attention to be paid to staff training at the time of induction, e.g. in-service training as a way of developing skills, team work and maintaining morale.

7 *Services for individuals.* District officers need to think and test out in advance systems for planning and monitoring the services designed for individual clients. This is one of the key features in the new service system and brings together issues of management, service planning and staff abilities when focusing on the needs of each client.

8 *The inevitability of mistakes.* Staff involved in the provision of new services need to be prepared for (and prepare others for – senior officers and DHA members) some mistakes. For example, incompatibilities will arise in living arrangements, clients may make additional demands on services, and officers must ensure that there is some slack in the services to be able to provide alternative arrangements where they are needed.

9 *Clients with special needs.* Planning services for individuals will begin to identify those clients who are, for a variety of reasons, likely to make greater demands on staff. There is a strong belief that some services ought to be provided early on for these clients, if only so that a district begins to gain some experience of how to do this well. The temptation is to leave these clients until last.

Hospital rundown

The Darenth Park Project cannot provide a blueprint for other hospital closures: each will differ because each will have a different history, traditions, culture, location, internal organization, and so on. But the problems each will face will largely be the same.

1 *Relations with new districts.* Both hospital managers and user district staff have strong obligations to keep each other fully informed of anything that is likely to affect the residents. This means that there must be clear lines of communication, agreed procedures for passing on information and authorized personnel with recognized status who speak for their organizations.

2 *Physical contraction.* Each hospital will want to close wards and reduce the amount of space used at the hospital as numbers of residents decline. Darenth Park planned and managed this itself and succeeded in some ways in minimizing the disruption caused to the residents. But by not involving district staff in this process, they may have missed an opportunity to regroup residents in relation to places of discharge.

3 *Redeployment of staff.* Staff should be made to feel from the beginning that there is a role for them to play in the new services if they want it. This requires an active programme of orientation towards a new philosophy of care (with user districts participating as well) and the positive encouragement of user districts to redeploy staff.

4 *Hospital maintenance.* All issues relating to the upkeep of the hospital should be looked at from the viewpoint of the client. It is important to continue to provide the same range of activities, especially social and recreational, until the hospital is finally closed.

5 *Residents' relations.* It is natural that the relatives of residents will turn first to ward staff for information on what will happen to their family member. Districts should be aware of this and should nominate one or two officers responsible for liaising with both ward staff and families over future plans and other issues of concern to families. The anxiety felt by families about such a change needs to be recognized and dealt with.

Finance

The arguments against community care have focused on two aspects. First, is the need for specialist facilities and services for some clients. Secondly, the extent to which these can be met depends on finance; community care cannot be seen as the cheap option. Good community care is costly. There are costs incurred in the transition phase as well as the funding already tied up in the hospital. We have shown how dependent most of the new services in the districts are on residents receiving social security funds. Threats to change the benefits system generate considerable uncertainty in the capacity of organizations to plan services effectively and to manage them if income levels vary. The staff in the districts see the major effort involved in creating a momentum in favour of community care, and, just when it looks as if it might succeed, the rules governing finance structure threaten to jeopardize this.

Normalization is not easy

In the districts, normalization became the driving force behind service provision, and one of the most instructive sets of lessons to come out of the Darenth Park Project has been how complex it is to implement policies based on the principles of normalization. Acquiring houses in the community is the easy part. What is much more difficult is knowing what to do with clients after that and having the capacity – in terms of finance, management and the right mix and numbers of professional staff – to be able to do it.

Normalization challenges the degree of control which both the NHS and social services have traditionally exercised over their own services and therefore over the clients who use those services. Clients are now seen at the centre of service provision, being encouraged to express views on how they see their needs and what they would like to happen. If they are not able to speak for themselves, advocacy schemes are being developed to ensure that the client's viewpoint is not lost. Many of the clients are now licensees of housing associations. Responsibility for the physical environment and to some extent for the well-being of clients is now shared with housing associations. Consortia may be involved, and they too share a concern over the quality of care offered to clients. Families may also take a greater interest in the type and adequacy of services on offer. It is now more widely recognized that many professions and agencies need to be involved.

It has not always been easy for districts to learn to share these responsibilities. All those who have an interest in the client need to participate early in the planning process, because otherwise they will not feel they have a stake in what happens. At the start of the Darenth Park Project, there was a tendency not to involve others in planning, on the grounds that this would cause delay, but the staff soon learned that it was not bringing in outside groups which caused delay, when plans had to be rethought and modified to meet the standards and wishes of others who had a legitimate stake. Sharing control resulted in more protracted planning but also resulted in smoother and speedier implementation and a more satisfactory role for clients and their families.

A second feature of new services is that clients should be able to exercise choice in all aspects of their lives. For this to be realistic, there needs to be a range of services available and also some slack built into the system so that choice is meaningful. Just as residential services have developed a wide variety of living arrangements, so day services are now beginning to see the need to diversify.

How realistic a choice have the Darenth Park residents had? In terms of where clients lived, in some districts choice was limited because there was only one type of facility being provided, i.e. group homes. Other districts had two or three types of accommodation. Individual placements were always made available where this seemed appropriate. Overall, for the 640 residents who were discharged from Darenth Park under the sponsorship of districts since 1983, there has been a fairly wide range of placements.

The range of day services has similarly varied across the districts. Some local authorities have been willing to make places available while others were not. ILEA has taken a strong interest in making educational provision for people with learning disabilities in further education colleges; other LEAs have offered less. Work training and employment opportunities have been the least developed of specifically organized day services. So for both residential and day-time activities, there is still some way to go before this objective is achieved.

Helping clients to learn how to choose is left to direct care staff, although it is up to the districts to indicate the importance attached to this activity. In almost all types of residential settings, it was very clear that staff were intensely proud of the progress their clients had made in learning how to choose what to wear, what to eat, when to go out, where to go and what to buy. In matters affecting their daily lives, through exercising choice, clients were beginning to develop a sense of themselves as individuals.

Integration is a third feature of normalization which districts claim to value – the use of existing community services and resources rather than the creation of special services and facilities for people with learning disabilities. Another aim of integration is for people with learning disabilities to spend time and have opportunities to mix socially and meet with people who do not have such disabilities. This requires a lot of work to make it happen. It involves sensitizing the providers of other community services to the needs of people with learning disabilities and may require supporting them as they learn how to approach and work with these clients. People with learning disabilities may also need to be shown how to use services.

The achievement of integration has been patchy so far. It is obvious that those clients who have the least disabilities have found it easiest to use community services and to devleop social contacts outside the home, usually through pubs and churches. Those factors which have prevented more integration include a lack of persistence by staff, or unawareness of community resources which might be appropriate; too few liaison staff to work with other agencies to familiarize them with the needs of people with learning disabilities; inadequate community facilities; and, occasionally, intolerance on the part of the public or professionals in the community. A further drawback is that many staff are young and not very well integrated in the community themselves. They may have moved to new locations to take up their jobs, and therefore have few local contacts to share with the clients.

Much has been done to see that people with learning disabilities use community facilities. However, much less has been done to ensure that they meet other members of the community on a social basis. Whatever the difficulties, integration must be kept as an objective if the policy is to work. There is something unsatisfactory about clients spending all their time with people who are paid to look after them. Care staff need to encourage friendships and focus on social activities as well as teaching clients to cook or use money. The government must recognize, too, that integration is difficult when clients have very little money to spend.

A fourth feature is privacy. It is now largely accepted that in people's homes single bedrooms will be provided unless clients specifically ask to share. The right to spatial privacy seems to be reasonably well accepted. But what about other forms of privacy? By not having relationships with people other than staff, clients in effect have no privacy from the staff; the staff know everything about what they do, who they speak to, what they say. By seeking planning permission for group homes, does not the principle of consultating on who may live where become a violation of privacy when particular clients move in?

The experience of the districts so far has shown how difficult it is, despite good intentions, to have a service function as it was intended to do. It requires a new management approach, which can share with others planning and provision and delivery of individual programmes of care. Regular monitoring of standards of care and assessment of residents' progress will be necessary. Staff working in dispersed and sometimes quite lonely situations need to be supported so that they do not become discouraged and so that they feel they can draw on others' experience to find ways of helping clients. And we need better methods of training staff so that they can perform the wide range of tasks now being expected of them. Staff should be able to meet regularly with those working in other group homes to share their experiences. In-service training and careful career planning will become necessary.

In many ways the task of sustaining the quality of the new services has barely begun.

Bibliography

Alaszewski, A. (1986). *Institutional Care and the Mentally Handicapped*. London, Croom Helm.

Anderson, M. (1971). *Family Structure in Nineteenth Century Lancashire*. Cambridge, Cambridge University Press.

Atkinson, D. (1988). Residential care for children and adults with mental handicap. In Wagner, Lady, *Report of a Committee on Residential Care*, Vol. 2. London, HMSO.

Audit Commission (1986). *Making a Reality of Community Care*. London, HMSO.

Audit Commission (1987). *Community Care: Developing Services for People with a Mental Handicap*. London, HMSO.

Barton, R. (1959). *Institutional Neurosis*. Bristol, John Wright.

Bayley, M. J. (1973). *Mental Handicap and Community Care*. London, Routledge and Kegan Paul.

Belknap, I. (1956). *Human Problems of a State Mental Hospital*. New York, McGraw-Hill.

Bella, D. A. (1976). Relationship of institutional size to quality of care. *American Journal of Mental Deficiency*, **81** (2), 117–23.

Bone, M., Spain, B. and Fox, M. (1972). *Plans and Provision for the Mentally Handicapped*. London, George Allen and Unwin.

Booth, T. (1985). *Home Truths*. London, Gower.

Braddock, D. and Heller, T. (1985). The closure of mental retardation institutions I & II. *Mental Retardation*, **23** (4), 168–76; **23** (5), 222–30.

Bradley, V. (1976). Policy termination in mental health: The hidden agenda! *Policy Sciences*, **7** (2), 215–24.

Brown, G. W., Bone, M., Dalison, B. and Wing, J. K. (1966). *Schizophrenia and Social Care*. Oxford, Oxford University Press.

Brown, P. (1985a). *The Transfer of Care: Psychiatric Deinstitutionalization and its Aftermath*. London, Routledge and Kegan Paul.

Brown, P. (ed.) (1985b). *Mental Health Care and Social Policy*. London, Routledge and Kegan Paul.

Cameron, J. M. (1978). Ideology and policy termination: Restructuring California's mental health system. *Public Policy*, **26** (4), 533–67.

Campaign for Mentally Handicapped People (1978). *ENCOR: A Way Ahead*. London, CMHP.

Cassell, W. A., Smith, C. M., Grunberg, F., Bean, J. and Thomas, R. (1972). Comparing costs of hospital and community based care. *Hospital and Community Psychiatry*, **23** (7).

Challis, L., Fuller, S., Henwood, M., Klein, R., Plowden, W., Webb, A., Whittingham, P. and Wistow, G. (1988). *Joint Approaches to Social Policy.* Cambridge, Cambridge University Press.

Chu, F. and Trotter, S. (1974). *The Madman Establishment: Ralph Nadar's Study Group Report on the National Institute of Mental Health.* New York, Grossman.

Conroy, J. W. and Bradley, V. J. (1985). *The Pennhurst Longitudinal Study: a Report of Five Years' Research and Analysis.* Philadelphia, Temple University.

Conroy, J., Efthimiou, J. and Lemanowicz, J. (1982). A matched comparison of the developmental growth of institutionalized and deinstitutionalized mentally retarded clients. *American Journal of Mental Deficiency,* **86** (6), 581–7.

Dalgleish, M. (1983). Assessment of residential environments for mentally retarded adults in Britain. *Mental Retardation,* **21** (5), 204–8.

Deutsch, A. (1940). *The Mentally Ill in America.* New York, Columbia University Press.

DHSS (1969). *Report of the Committee of Enquiry into the Allegations of Ill Treatment and other Irregularities at the Ely Hospital, Cardiff.* Cmnd. 3975. London, HMSO.

DHSS (1970). *Reorganising the National Health Service.* London, HMSO.

DHSS (1971). *Better Services for the Mentally Handicapped.* Cmnd. 4683. London, HMSO.

DHSS (1975). *Better Services for the Mentally Ill.* Cmnd. 6233. London, HMSO.

DHSS (1976). *Priorities for Health and Personal Social Services.* London, HMSO.

DHSS (1977). *Joint Care Planning: Health and Local Authorities.* HC(77)17 and LAC(77)10. London, HMSO.

DHSS (1978). *Report of the Committee of Enquiry into Normansfield Hospital.* Cmnd. 7357. London, HMSO.

DHSS (1979). *A Report of the Committee of Enquiry into Mental Handicap Nursing and Care* (Jay Report). Cmnd. 7468. London, HMSO.

DHSS (1980). *Mental Handicap: Progress, Problems, and Priorities.* London, DHSS.

DHSS (1981a). *Care in Action.* Cmnd. 8173. London, HMSO.

DHSS (1981b). *Care in the Community: A Consultative Document for Moving Resources for Care in England.* HC(81)9, LAC(81)5. London, DHSS.

DHSS (1981c). *Report on Community Care.* London, HMSO.

DHSS (1981d). *Growing Older.* Cmnd. 8173. London, HMSO.

DHSS (1983a). *NHS Management Enquiry Report* (Griffiths Report). London, HMSO.

DHSS (1983b). *Care in the Community.* HC(83)6 and LAC(83)5. London, HMSO.

DHSS (1983c). *Getting Mentally Handicapped Children Out of Hospital.* DA(83)3. London, HMSO.

DHSS (1984). *Health Services Development: Collaboration between NHS, Local Government and Voluntary Organisations.* HC(84)9. London, HMSO.

DHSS (1985). *Government Response to the Second Report from the Special Services Committee 1984–85 Session: Community Care.* Cmnd. 9674. London, HMSO.

DHSS (1987). *Option Appraisal: A Guide for the NHS.* London, HMSO.

DHSS (1988). *Community Care: Agenda for Action.* London, HMSO.

DOE (1988). *Policy Planning Guidance: Green Belt Land.* London, HMSO.

Dunham, H. W. and Weinberg, S. K. (1960). *The Culture of the State Mental Hospital.* Detroit, Wayne State University Press.

Dunleavy, P. (1987). *Democracy, the State and Public Choice.* Brighton, Wheatsheaf.

Endicott, J., Hertz, M. and Gibbon, M. (1978). Brief versus standard hospitalization: the differential costs. *American Journal of Psychiatry,* **135** (6).

Estes, C., Newcomer, R. J. and Associates (1983). *Fiscal Austerity and Aging.* Beverly Hills, Calif., Sage.

Evans, G., Todd, S., Blunden, R., Porterfield, J. and Ager, A. (1987). Evaluation: the impact of a move to ordinary housing. *British Journal of Subnormality*, **33** (1), 10–18.

Fenton, J. R., Tessier, L., Contandinopoulas, A. P., Nguyer, A. and Struening, E. L. (1982). A comparative trial of home and hospital psychiatric treatment: financial costs. *Canadian Journal of Psychiatry*, **27** (3).

Freeman, H. and Farndale, J. (eds) (1963). *Trends in the Mental Health Services*. Oxford, Pergamon Press.

Friend, J. K., Power, J. M. and Yewlett, C. J. (1974). *Public Planning: The Inter Corporate Dimension*. London, Tavistock.

Glennerster, H., Korman, N. and Marsden-Wilson, F. (1983). *Planning for Priority Groups*. Oxford, Blackwell.

Goffman, E. (1961). *Asylum: Essays on the Social Situation of Mental Patients and Other Inmates*. New York, Doubleday.

Greenblatt, M., York, R. and Brown, E. (1955). *From Custodial to Therapeutic Patient Care in Mental Hospitals*. New York, Russell Sage Foundation.

Grob. G. N. (1983). *Mental Illness and American Society, 1875–1940*. Princeton, Princeton University Press.

Hoult, J., Reynolds, I., Charboneau-Powis, M., Weekes, P. and Briggs, J. (1983). Psychiatric hospital versus community treatment: the results of a randomised trial. *Australian and New Zealand Journal of Psychiatry*, **17**, 160–7.

House of Commons (1985). Second Report of the Social Services Committee, *Community Care*. HC.13. London, HMSO.

Jay Committee (1979). *A Report of the Committee of Enquiry into Mental Handicap Nursing and Care*, Cmnd. 7468. London, HMSO.

Jeffrae, D. and Cheseldine, S. (1982). *Pathways to Independence*. Sevenoaks, Hodder and Stoughton Educational.

Jones, K. (1960). *Mental Health and Social Policy 1845–1959*. London, Routledge and Kegan Paul.

Jones, K. (1972). *A History of the Mental Health Services*. London, Routledge and Kegan Paul.

Jones, K. and Fowles, A. J. (1984). *Ideas on Institutions: Analysing the Literature on Long Term Care and Custody*. London, Routledge and Kegan Paul.

Jones, K. with Brown, J., Cunningham, W. J., Roberts, J. and Williams, P. (1975). *Opening the Door: A Study of New Policies for the Mentally Handicapped*. London, Routledge and Kegan Paul.

King, R. D., Raynes, N. V. and Tizard, J. (1971). *Patterns of Residential Care: Sociological Studies in Institutions for Handicapped Children*. London, Routledge and Kegan Paul.

King's Fund Centre (1980). *An Ordinary Life*. London, King's Fund Centre.

Knapp, M. and Beecham, J. (1989). *The Cost-effectiveness of Community Care for Former Long Stay Psychiatric Hospital Patients*, Discussion Paper No. 533/2, Canterbury, PSSRU University of Kent.

Knapp, M., Beecham, J. and Renshaw, J. (1987). *The Cost Effectiveness of Psychiatric Reprovision Services*. PSSRU Discussion Paper 533/2. University of Kent, Canterbury.

Korman, N. and Glennerster, H. (1985). *Closing a Hospital: The Darenth Park Project*. Occasional Papers in Social Administration, No. 78. London, Bedford Square Press.

Leedham, I. (1988). *Output Evaluation in Practice: Research Methodology with Special Reference to Services for People with Learning Difficulties*. Discussion paper 606/2, Personal Social Services Research Unit, University of Kent at Canterbury.

Lindblom, C. (1965). *The Intelligence of Democracies*. New York, Free Press.

Locker, D., Rao, B. and Weddell, J. M. (1984). Evaluating community care for the mentally handicapped adult: a comparison of hostel, home and hospital care. *Journal of Mental Deficiency Research*, **28**, 189–98.

MacEachron, A. E. (1983). Institutional reform and adaptive functioning of mentally retarded persons: a field experiment. *American Journal of Mental Deficiency*, **88** (1), 2–12.

Martin, J. (1984). *Hospitals in Trouble*. Oxford, Blackwell.

Mayer, J. A. (1983). Notes towards a working definition of social control in historical analysis. In Cohen, S. and Scull, A. J. (eds), *Social Control and the State*. Oxford, Martin Robertson.

McDonagh, O. (1960). *A Pattern of Government Growth: The Passenger Acts and their Enforcement*. London, MacGibbon and Key.

Ministry of Health (1962). *A Hospital Plan for England and Wales*. Cmnd. 1604. London, HMSO.

Morris, P. (1969). *Put Away: A Sociological Study of Institutions for the Mentally Retarded*. London, Routledge and Kegan Paul.

Mueller, D. C. (1979). *Public Choice*. Cambridge, Cambridge University Press.

National Audit Office (1987). *Community Care Development*. London, HMSO.

National Council for Civil Liberties (1951). *50,000 Outside the Law*. London, NCCL.

National Development Group for the Mentally Handicapped (1976). *Mental Handicap: Planning Together*. London, HMSO.

National Development Group for the Mentally Handicapped (1977). *Mentally Handicapped Children. A Plan for Action*. London, HMSO.

National Development Group for the Mentally Handicapped (1980). *Services for Mentally Handicapped People – Unfinished Business*. London, DHSS.

New Concepts for the Handicapped Inc. (1982). *Getting to Know You*. Wisconsin, distributed in the UK by CMH.

Niskanen, W. (1971). *Bureaucracy and Representative Government*. Chicago, Aldine Atherton.

O'Connor, N. and Tizard, J. (1956). *The Social Problems of Mental Deficiency*. Oxford, Pergamon Press.

O'Donnell, O., Maynard, A. and Wright, K. (1988). *The Economic Evaluation of Mental Health Care: A Review*. Discussion Paper No. 51. University of York, Centre for Health Economics.

Oswin, M. (1974). *The Empty Hours*. Harmondsworth, Penguin.

Parker, R. (1988). An historical background to residential care. In Wagner, Lady, *Report of a Committee on Residential Care*, Vol. 2. London, HMSO.

Peters, T. S. and Waterman, R. H. (1982). *In Search of Excellence: Lessons from America's Best Run Companies*. New York, Harper and Row.

Pratt, M. W., Luszcz, M. A. and Brown, M. E. (1980). Measuring dimensions of the quality of care in small community residences. *American Journal of Mental Deficiency*, **85** (2), 188–94.

Race, D. G. and Race, D. M. (1979). *The Cherries Group Home: A Beginning*. London, HMSO.

Ramon, S. (1985). *Psychiatry in Britain: Meaning and Policy*. London, Croom Helm.

Robb, B. (1967). *Sans Everything*. London, Nelson.

Rochester, C. (1987). *Southwark Consortium (1984–87)*. Unpublished report to Cambridge House.

Saxby, H., Thomas, M., Felce, D. and De Kock, U. (1986). The use of shops, cars and public houses by severely and profoundly mentally handicapped adults. *British Journal of Mental Subnormality*, **32** (2), 69–81.

Schalock, R. L. and Lilley, M. A. (1986). Placement from community-based mental retardation programs: how well do clients do after 8 to 10 years? *American Journal of Mental Deficiency*, **90** (6), 669–76.

Scull, A. (1979). *Museums of Madness: The Social Organisation of Insanity in 19th Century England*. London, Allen Lane.

Scull, A. (1984). *Decarceration: Community Treatment and the Deviant – A Radical View*, 2nd edn. New Jersey, Rugers University Press.

Sedgwick, P. (1982). *Psycho-Politics*. New York, Harper and Row.

Segal, S. P. and Aviram, V. (1978). *The Mentally Ill in Community-based Sheltered Care*. New York, John Wiley.

Sheehan, D. M. and Atkinson, J. (1974). Comparative costs of state hospital and community based inpatients case in Texas: Who benefits most? *Hospital and Community Psychiatry*, **25**, 242–4.

Sheill, A. and Wright, K. (1988). *Counting the Cost of Community Care*. York, Centre for Health Economics.

Skultans, V. (1978). *English Madness: Ideas on Insanity 1580–1890*. London, Routledge and Kegan Paul.

Smith, J., Glossop, C. and Kushlick, A. (1980). Evaluation of alternative residential facilities of the severely mentally handicapped in Wessex: client progress. *Advances in Behaviour Research and Therapy*, **3**, 5–11.

Stanton, A. H. and Schwarz, M. S. (1954). *The Mental Hospital*. New York, Basic Books.

Thomas, M., Felce, D., De Kock, U., Saxby, H. and Repp, A. (1986). The activity of staff and of severely and profoundly mentally handicapped adults in residential settings of different sizes. *British Journal of Mental Subnormality*, **32** (1), 82–92.

Thompson, T. and Carey, A. (1980). Structured normalization: intellectual and adaptive behavior changes in a residential setting. *Mental Retardation*, **18** (4), 193–7.

Titmuss, R. M. (1963). Community care: Fact or fiction. In Freeman, H. and Farndale, J. (eds), *Trends in the Mental Health Services*. Oxford, Pergamon Press.

Tizard, J. (1964). *Community Services for the Mentally Handicapped*. Oxford, Oxford University Press.

Tizard, J. and Grad, J. C. (1961). *The Mentally Handicapped and their Families: A Social Survey*. Oxford, Oxford University Press.

Townsend, P. (1962). *The Last Refuge*. London, Routledge and Kegan Paul.

Tredgold, A. (1908). *Mental Deficiency*. London, Ballière Tyndale.

Tyerman, C. and Spencer, C. (1980). Normalised physical environment for the mentally handicapped and its effects on patterns of activity, social relations and self-help skills. *British Journal of Mental Subnormality*, **26** (50), 47–54.

Tyne, A. (1982). Community care and mentally handicapped people. In Walker, A. (ed.), *Community Care: The Family, the State and Social Policy*. Oxford, Blackwell.

Wagner, Lady (1988). *Report of a Committee on Residential Care*, Vol. 2. London, HMSO.

Walker, A. (ed.) (1982). *Community Care: The Family, the State and Social Policy*. Oxford, Blackwell.

Weisbrod, B. A. *et al.* (1980). Alternatives to mental hospital treatment: 1 economic benefit-cost analysis. *Archives of General Psychiatry*, **32**, 400–5.

Wertheimer, A. (1986). Mental handicap: Where do they go from here? *Mental Handicap Bulletin*, **61** (2).

Willcocks, D., Peace, S. and Kellaherr, L. (1987). *Private Lives in Public Places*. London, Tavistock.

Wing, L. (1984). *Annual Report for the DHSS*. London, MRC Social Psychiatry Research Unit.

Wing, L. (1989). *Hospital Closure and the Resettlement of Residents: The Case of Darenth Park*. Aldershot, Gower.

Witt, S. J. (1981). Increase in adaptive behavior level after residence in an intermediate care facility for mentally retarded persons. *Mental Retardation*, **19** (2), 75–9.

Wolfensberger, W. (1972). *The Principle of Normalisation in Human Services.* Toronto, National Institute on Mental Retardation.

Wright, K. (1987). *Cost Effectiveness in Community Care.* Discussion Paper No. 33. University of York, Centre for Health Economics.

Wright, K. and Haycox, A. (1984). *Public Sector Costs of Caring for Mentally Handicapped Persons in a Large Hospital.* Discussion Paper No. 1. University of York, Centre for Health Economics.

Wright, K. and Haycox, A. (1985). *Costs of Alternative Forms of NHS Care for Mentally Handicapped Persons.* Discussion Paper No. 7. University of York, Centre for Health Economics.

Index

This book is to be returned on or before
d below.

WITHDRAWN

SOCIAL SCIENCE LIBRARY

Manor Road Building
Manor Road
Oxford OX1 3UQ
Tel: (2)71093 (enquiries and renewals)
http://www.ssl.ox.ac.uk

This is a NORMAL LOAN item.

We will email you a reminder before this item is due.

Please see http://www.ssl.ox.ac.uk/lending.html
for details on:

- loan policies; these are also displayed on the
  notice boards and in our library guide.

- how to check when your books are due back.

- how to renew your books, including information
  on the maximum number of renewals.
  Items may be renewed if not reserved by
  another reader. Items must be renewed before
  the library closes on the due date.

- level of fines; fines are charged on overdue books.

Please note that this item may be recalled during Term.

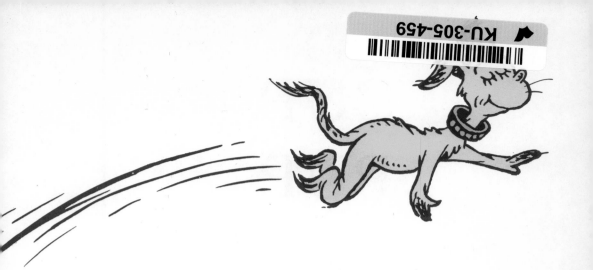

UP
PUP

Pup is up.

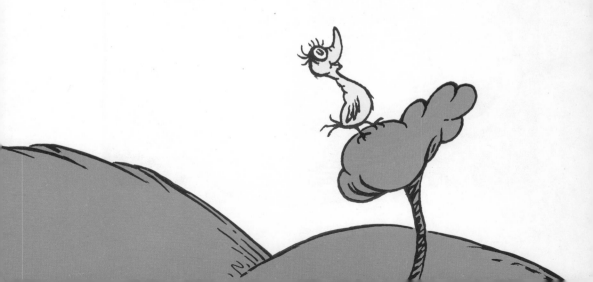

CUP
PUP

Pup in cup

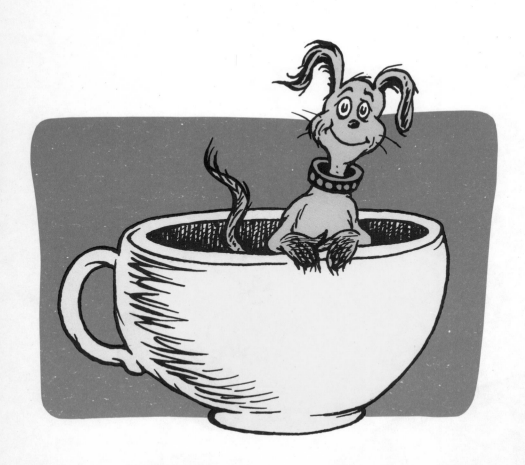

HOP

Warwickshire County Council

This item is to be returned or renewed before the latest date above. It may be borrowed for a further period if not in demand. **To renew your books:**

- **Phone the 24/7 Renewal Line 01926 499273 or**
- **Visit www.warwickshire.gov.uk/libraries**

Discover • Imagine • Learn • *with libraries*

Warwickshire County Council

Working for Warwickshire

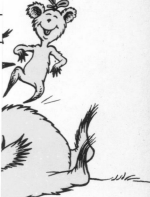

By Dr. Seuss

CO

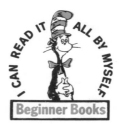

Trademark of Random House, Inc., William Collins Sons & Co. Ltd., Authorised User

CONDITIONS OF SALE
The paperback edition of this book is sold subject to the
condition that it shall not, by way of trade or otherwise,
be lent, re-sold, hired out or otherwise circulated without
the publisher's prior consent in any form of binding or
cover other than that in which it is published and without
a similar condition including this condition being imposed
on the subsequent purchaser.

6 7 8 9 10

ISBN 0 00 171309 4 (paperback)
ISBN 0 00 171118 0 (hardback)

© 1963 by Dr. Seuss
A Beginner Book Published by arrangement with
Random House, Inc., New York, New York
First published in Great Britain 1964

Printed in Hong Kong

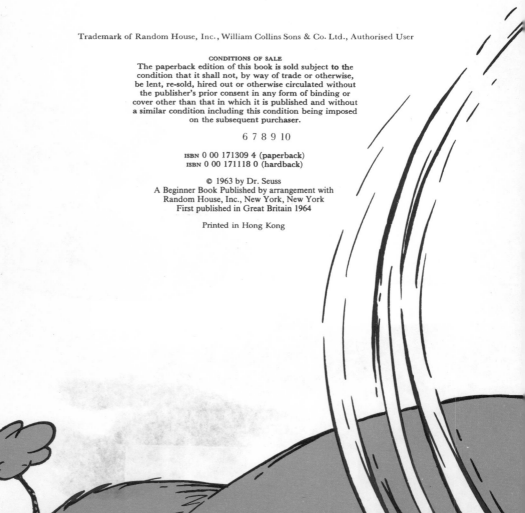

PUP
CUP

Cup on pup

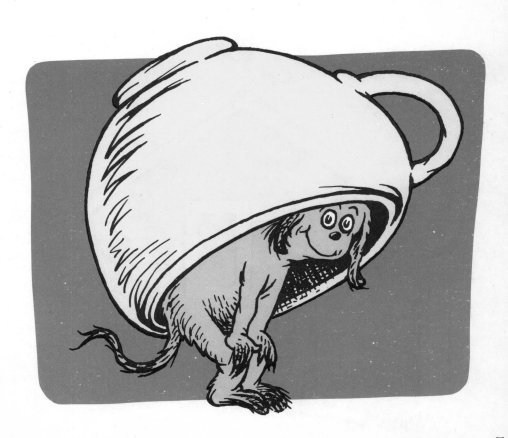

MOUSE
HOUSE

Mouse on house

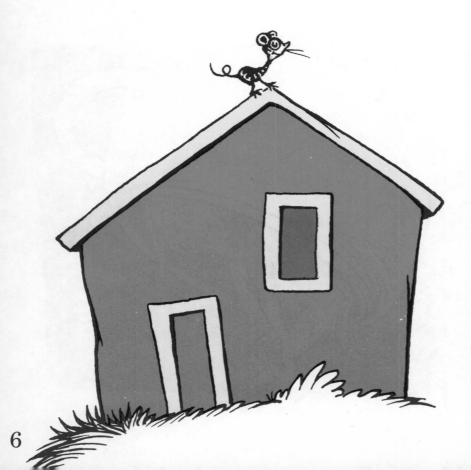

HOUSE
MOUSE

House on mouse

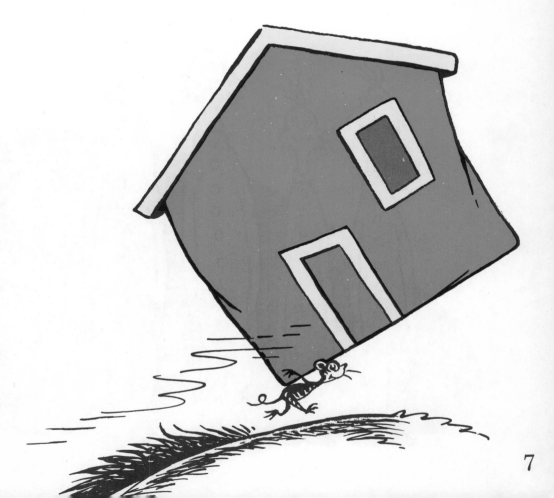

ALL
TALL

We all are tall.

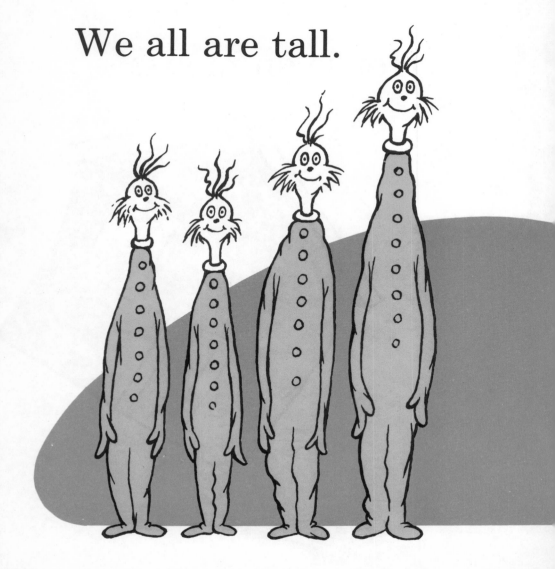

ALL
SMALL

We all are small.

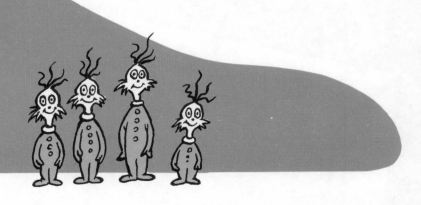

ALL
BALL

We all play ball

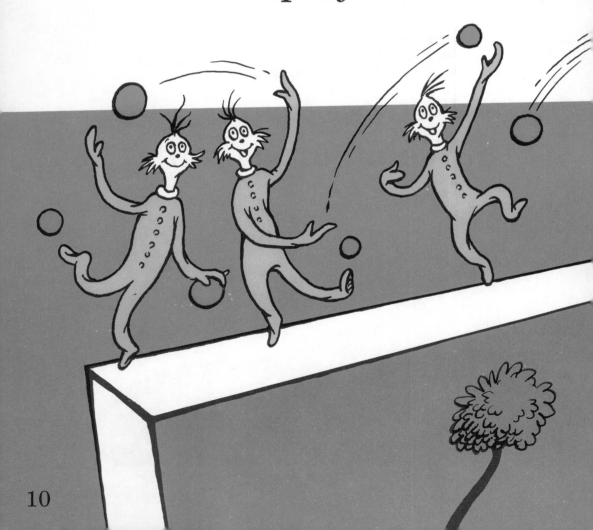

BALL
WALL

up on a wall.

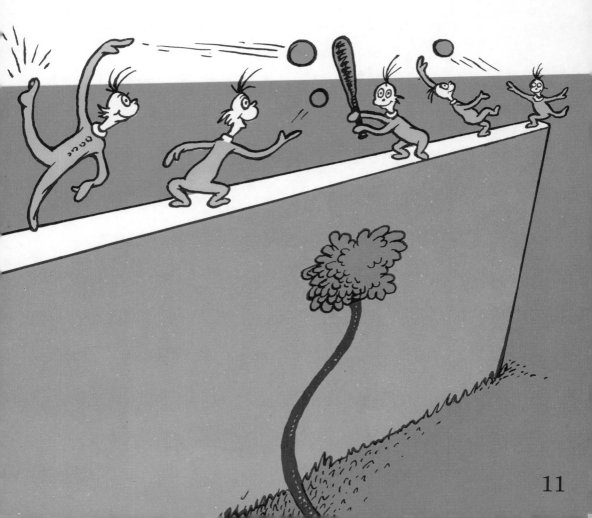

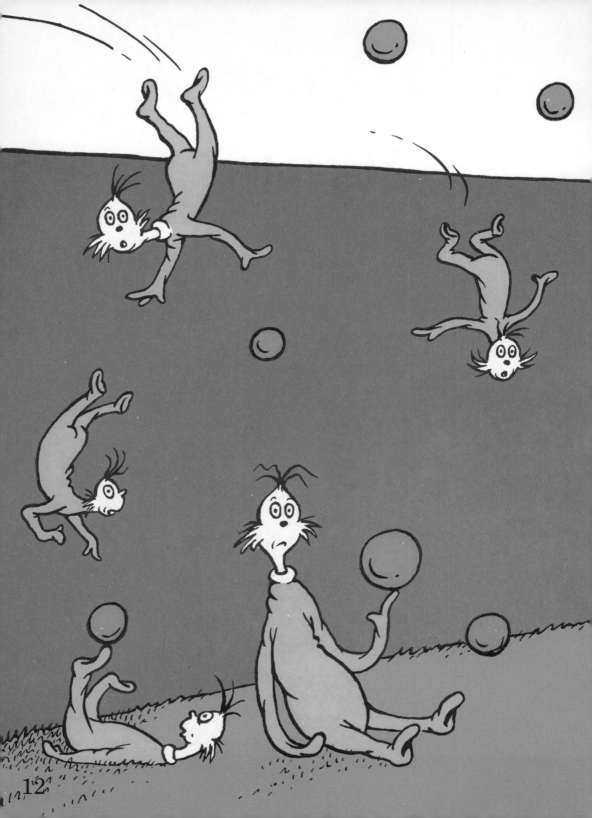

12

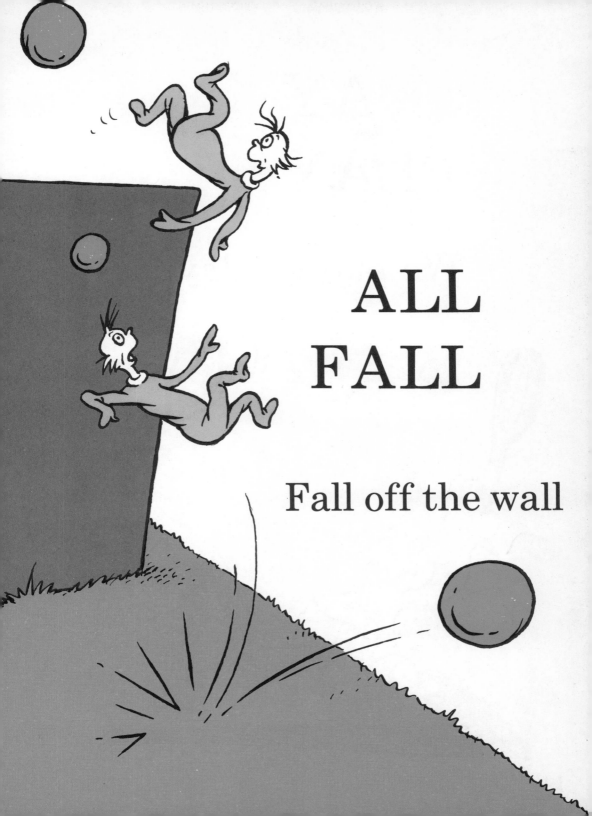

ALL
FALL

Fall off the wall

DAY
PLAY

We play all day.

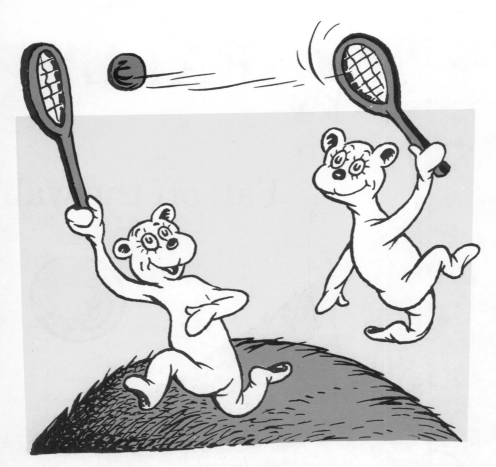

NIGHT
FIGHT

We fight all night.

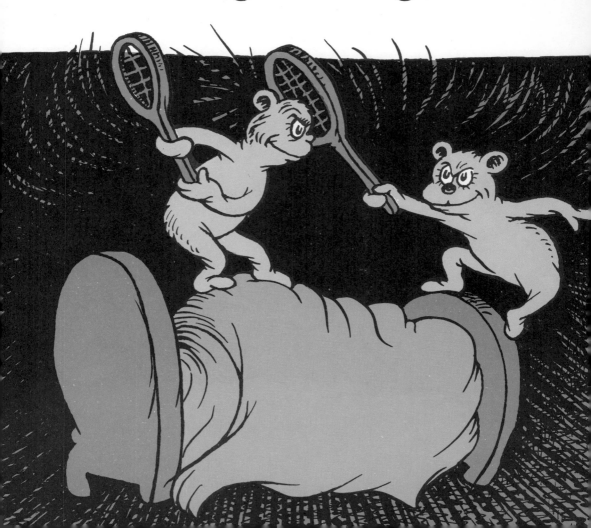

HE
ME

He is after me.

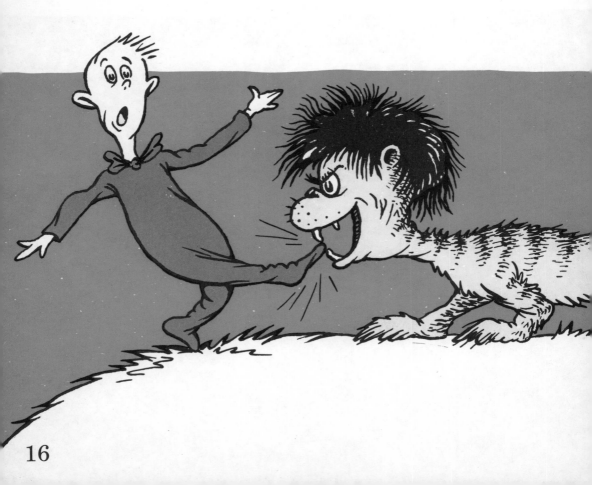

HIM
JIM

Jim is after him.

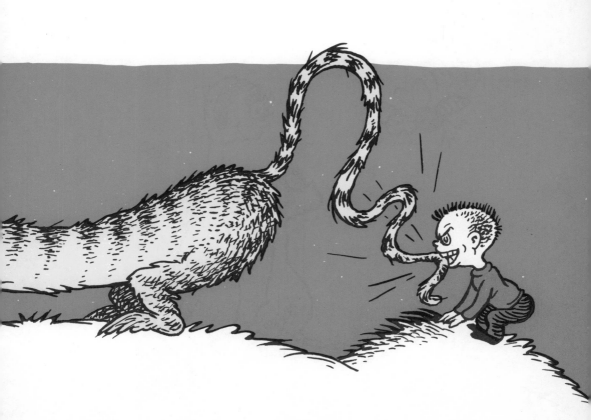

SEE
BEE

We see a bee.

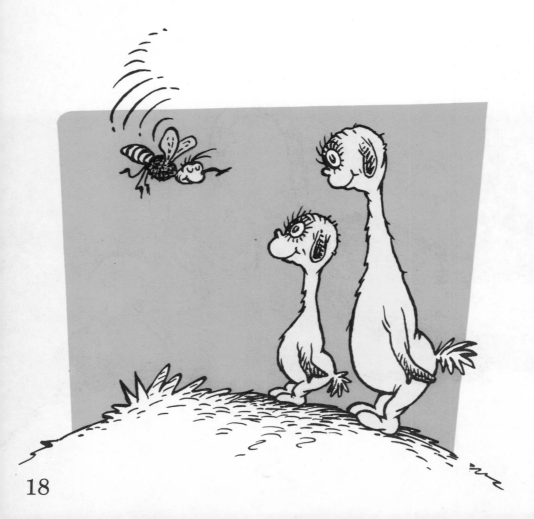

SEE
BEE
THREE

Now we
see three.

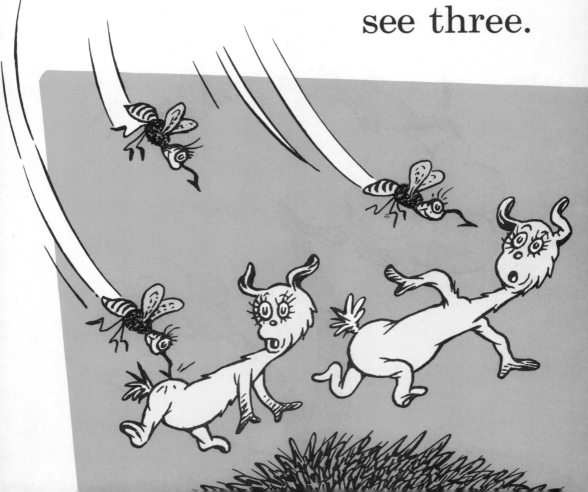

THREE
TREE

Three fish in a tree

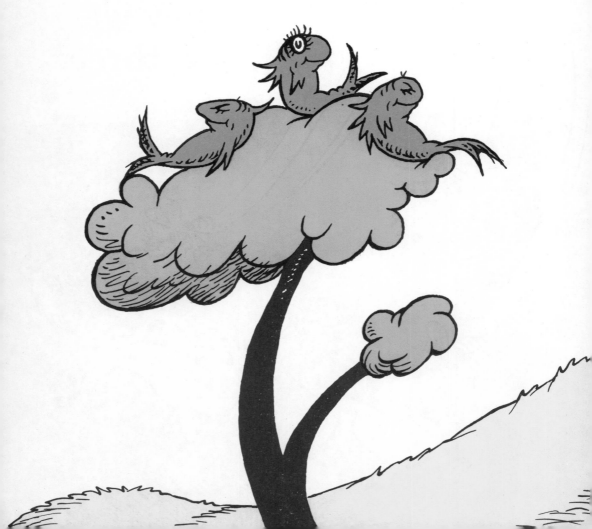

Fish in a tree?
How can that be?

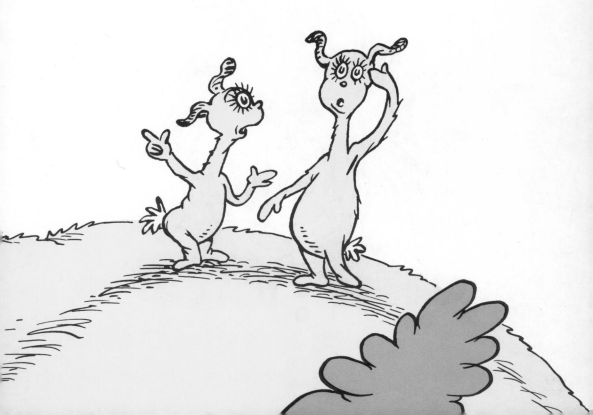

RED
RED

They call me Red.

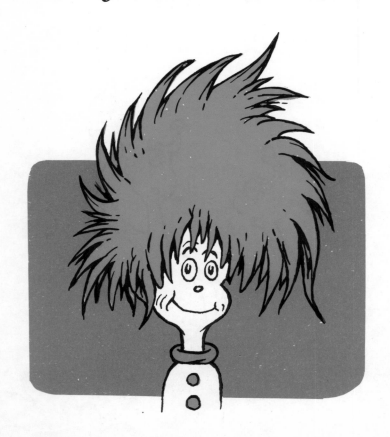

RED
BED

I am in bed.

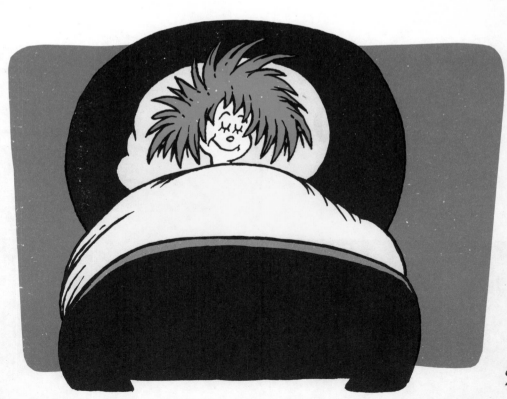

RED
NED
TED
and
ED
in
BED

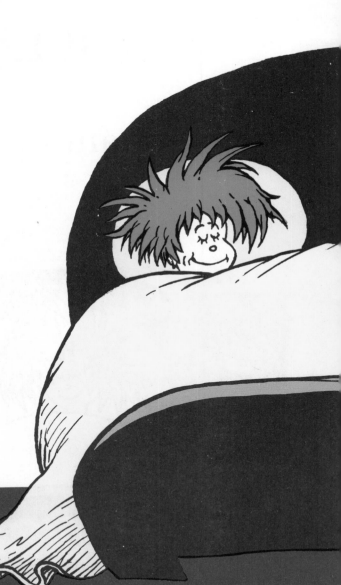

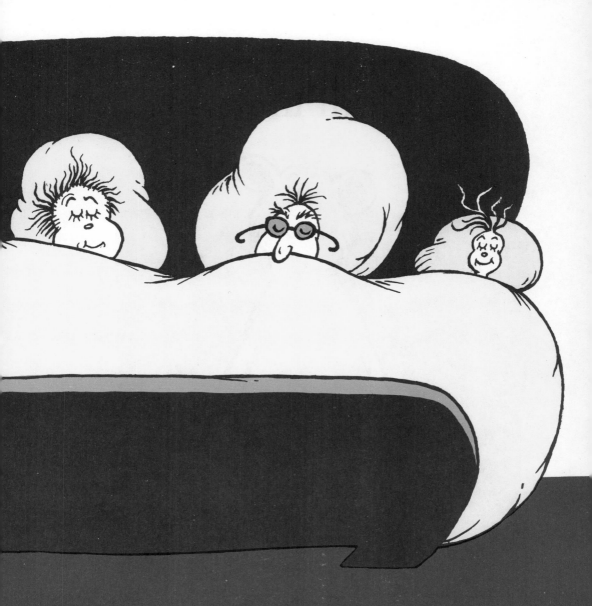

PAT
PAT

They call him Pat.

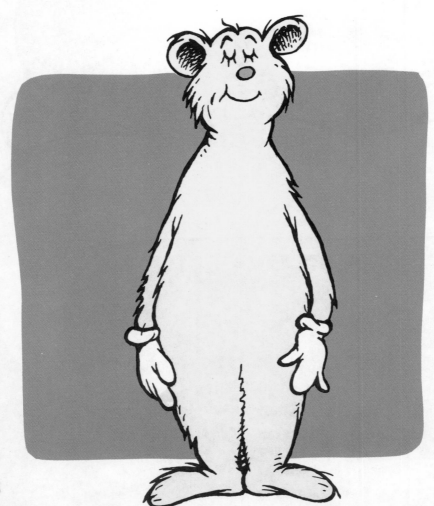

PAT
SAT

Pat sat on hat.

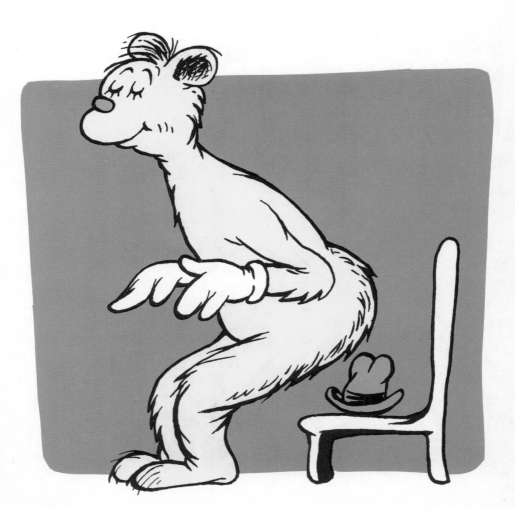

PAT
CAT

Pat sat on cat.

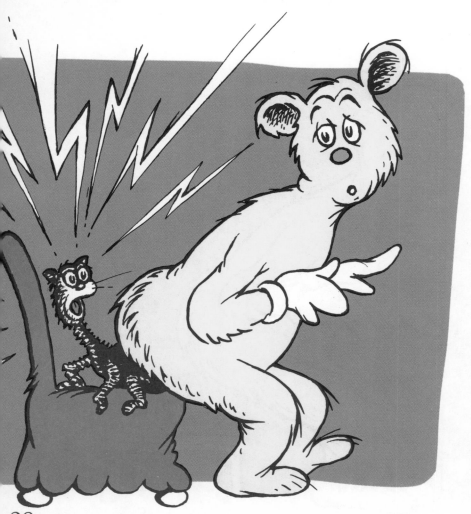

PAT
BAT

Pat sat on bat.

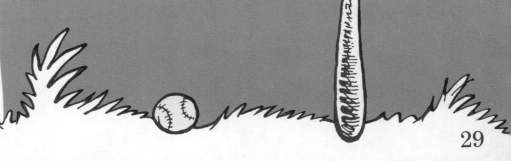

NO
PAT
NO

Don't sit on that.

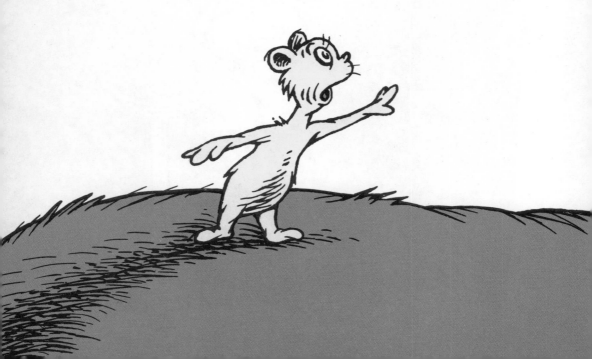

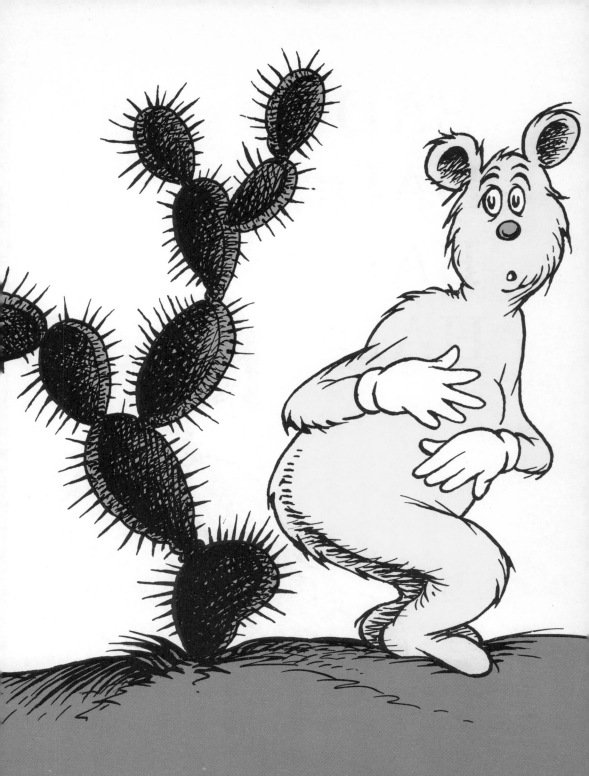

SAD

DAD

BAD

HAD

Dad is sad
very, very sad.
He had a bad day.
What a day Dad had!

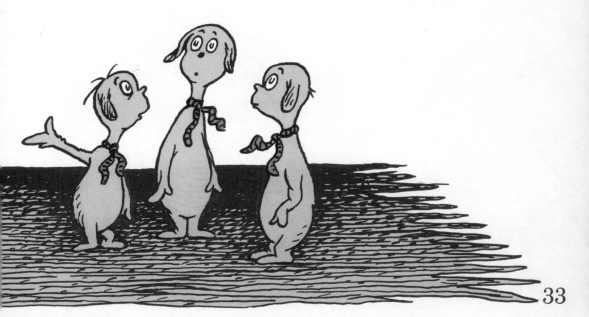

THING
THING

What is that thing?

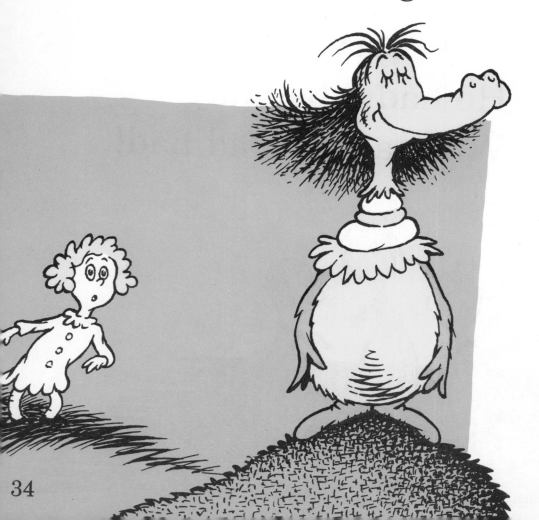

THING
SING

That thing can sing!

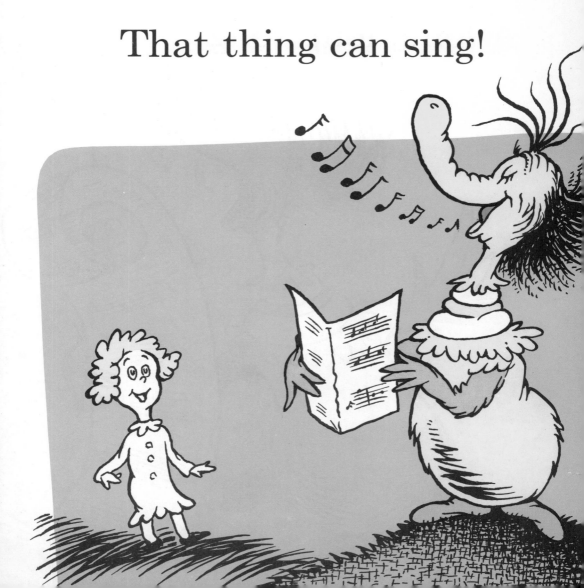

SONG
LONG

A long, long song

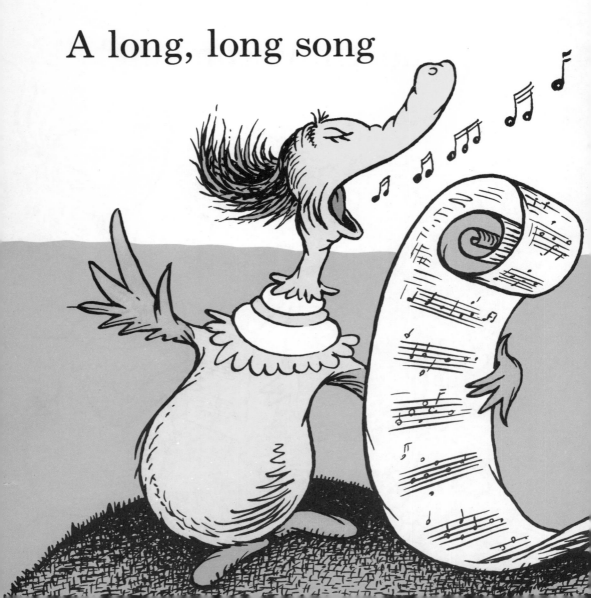

Good-by, Thing.
You sing too long.

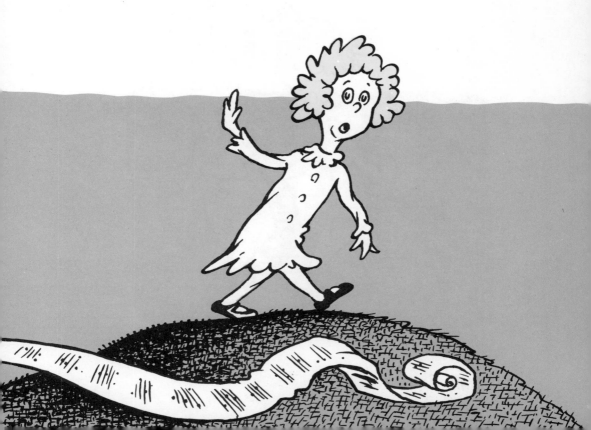

WALK
WALK

We like to walk.

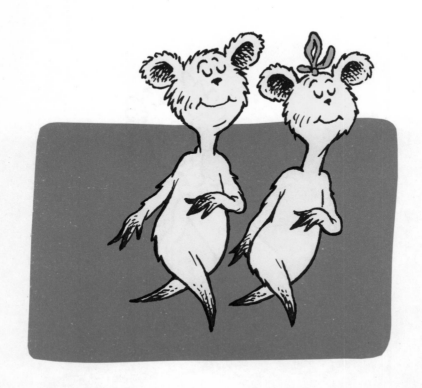

WALK
TALK

We like to talk.

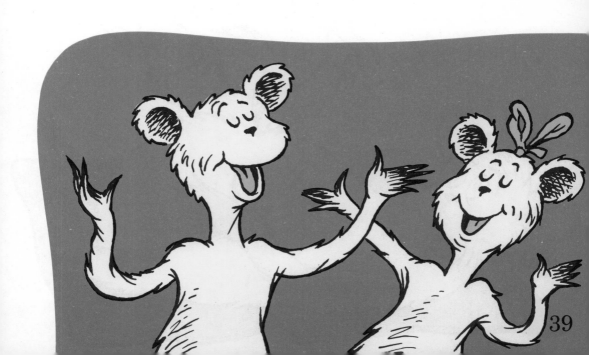

39

HOP
POP

We like to hop.
We like to hop
on top of Pop.

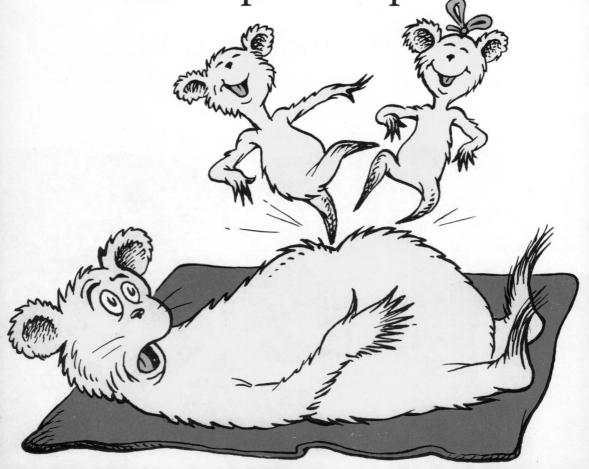

STOP

You must not
hop on Pop.

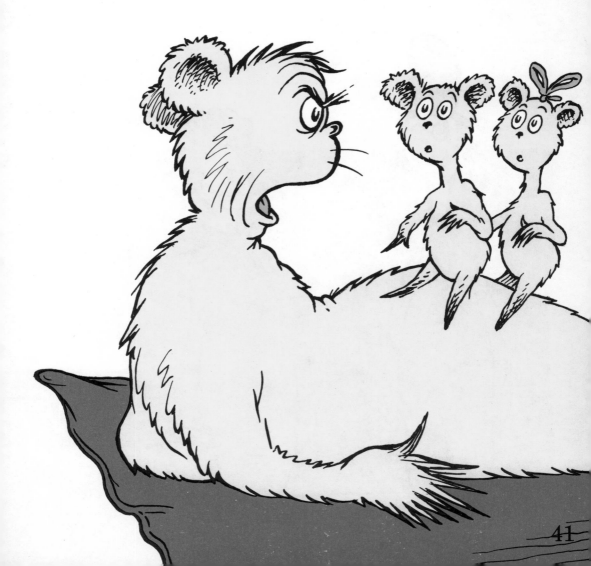

Mr. BROWN
Mrs. BROWN

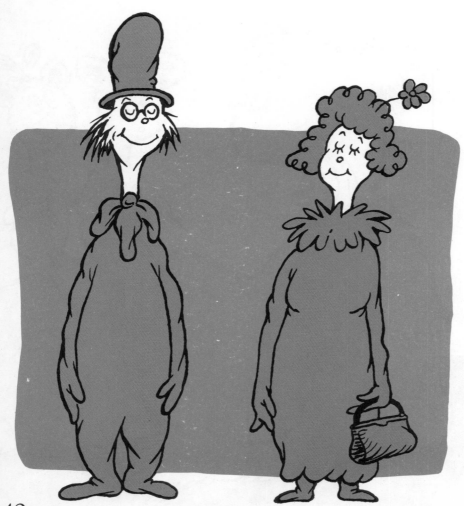

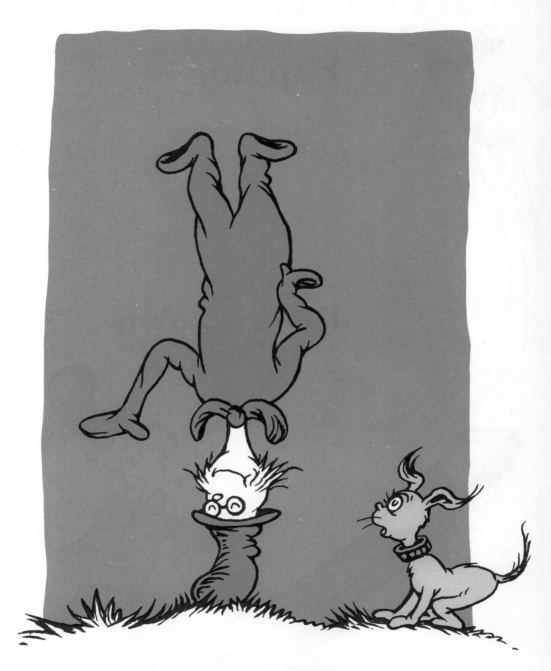

Mr. Brown upside down

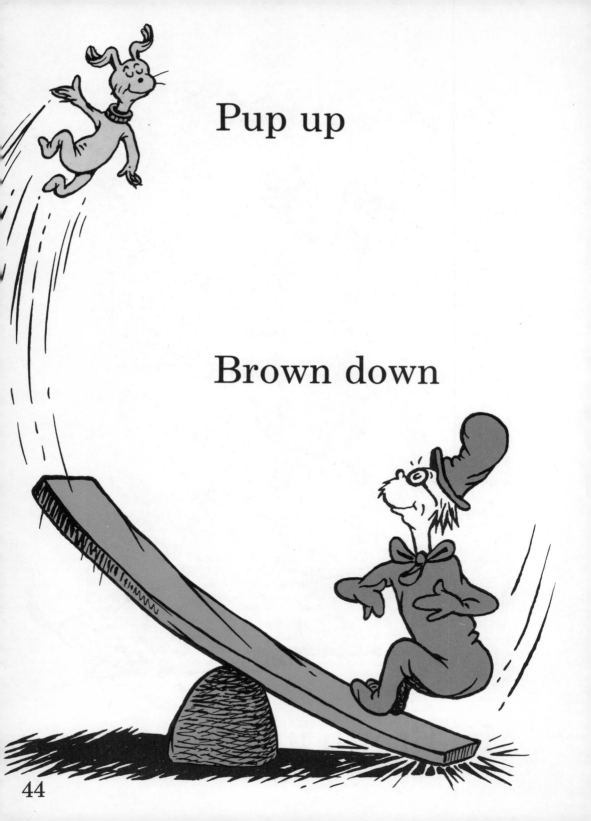

Pup up

Brown down

44

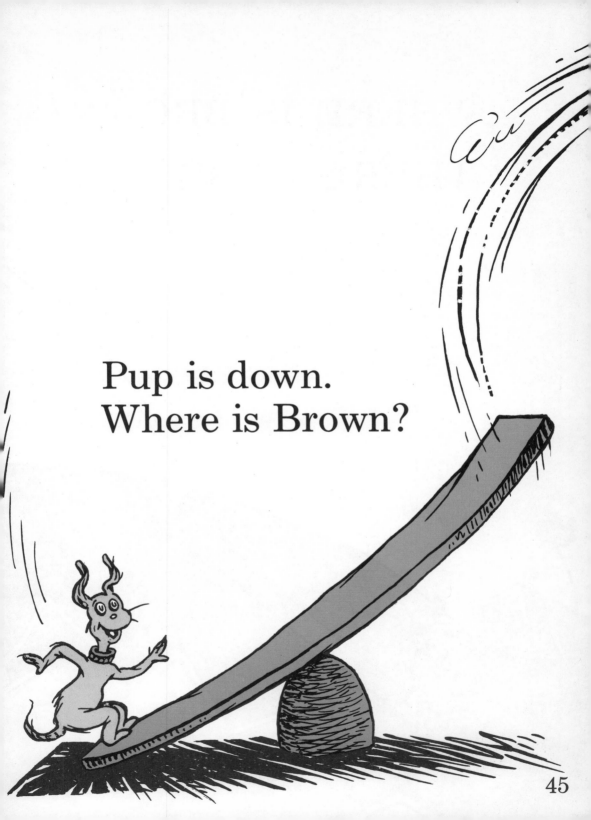

Pup is down.
Where is Brown?

WHERE IS BROWN?
THERE IS BROWN!

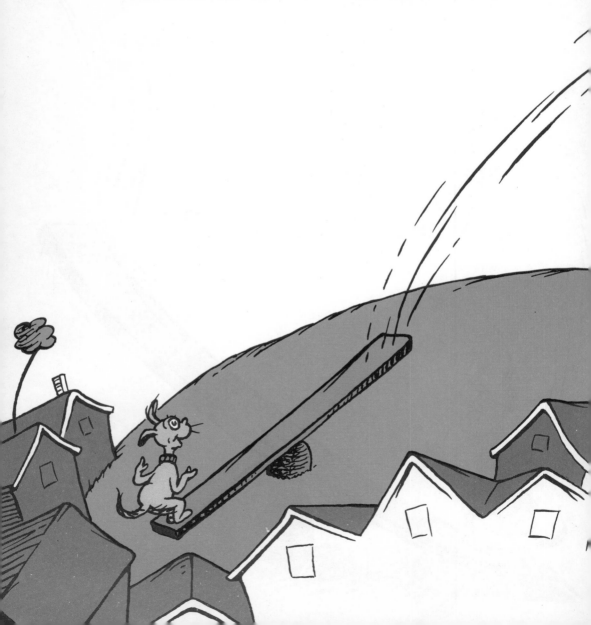

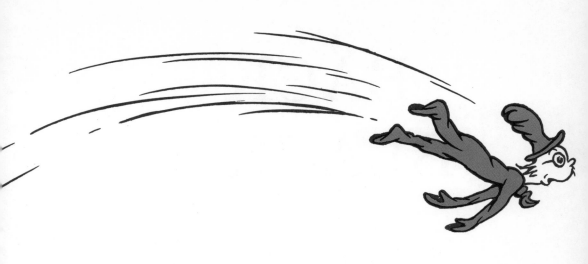

Mr. Brown is out of town.

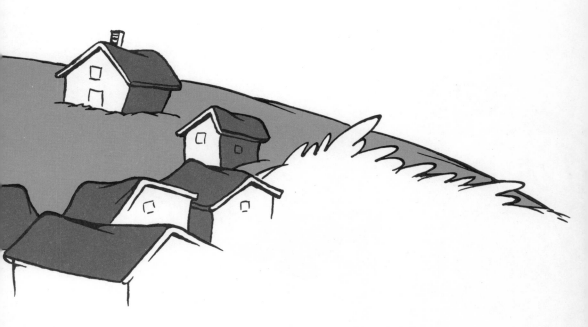

BACK
BLACK

Brown came back.

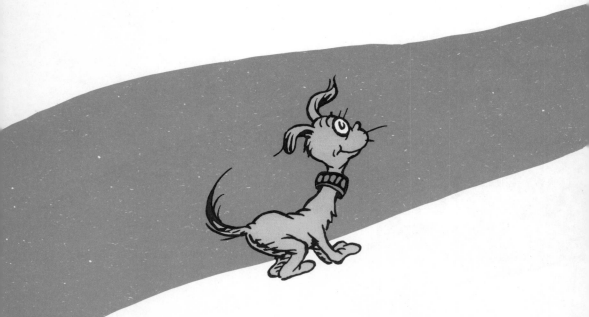

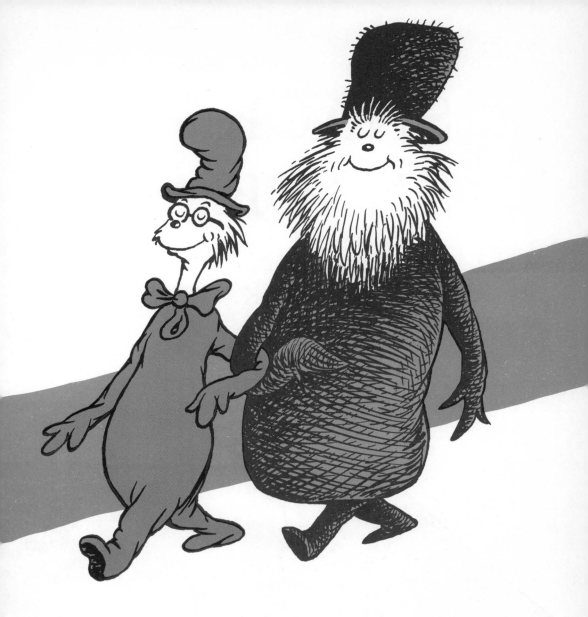

Brown came back
with Mr. Black.

SNACK SNACK

Eat a snack.

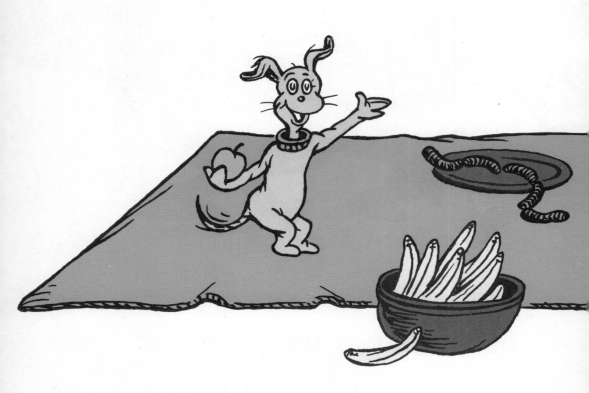

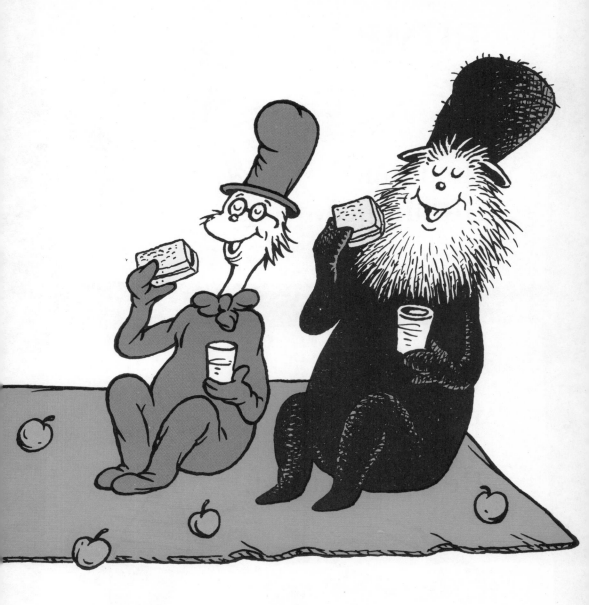

Eat a snack
with Brown and Black.

JUMP
BUMP

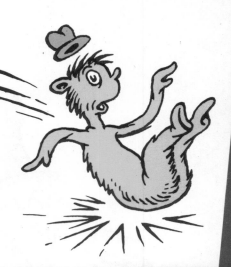

He jumped.
He bumped.

FAST
PAST

He went past fast.

WENT
TENT
SENT

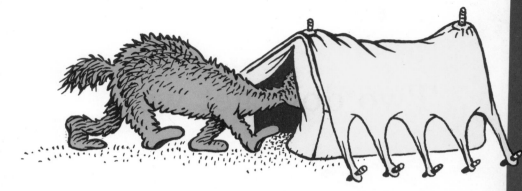

He went into the tent.

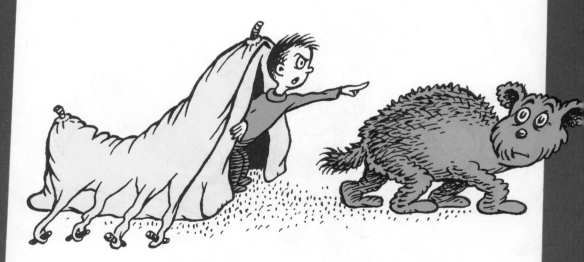

I sent him out of the tent.

WET
GET

Two dogs get wet.

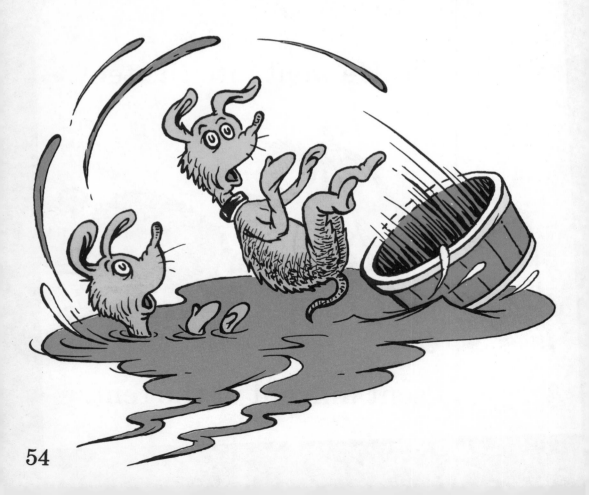

HELP
YELP

They yelp for help.

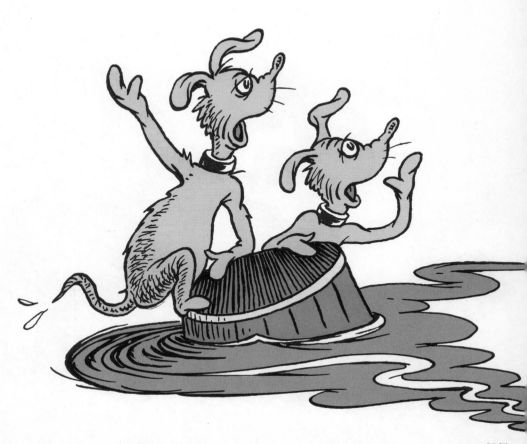

HILL
WILL

Will went up the hill.

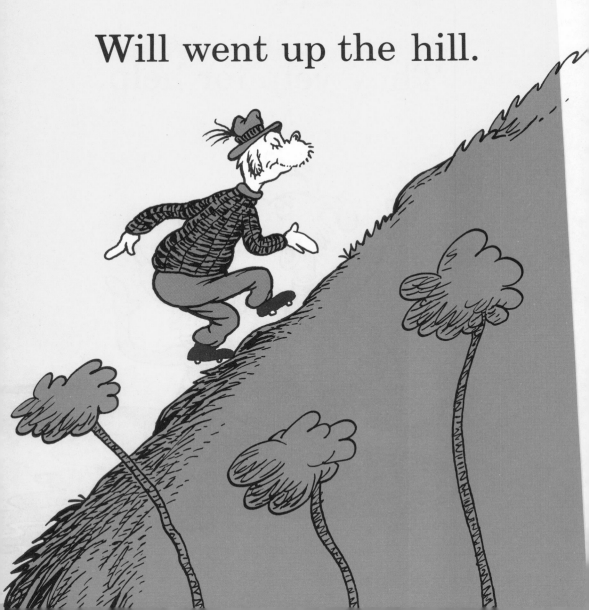

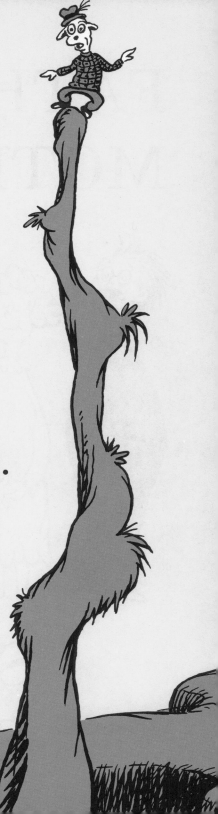

WILL
HILL
STILL

Will is
up the hill still.

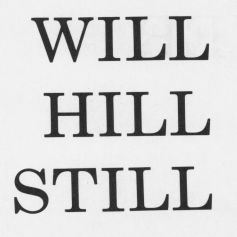

FATHER
MOTHER

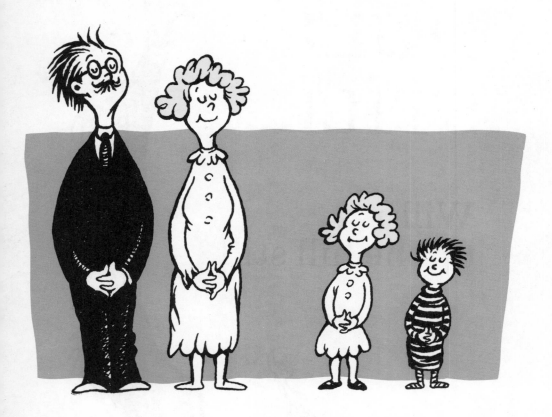

SISTER
BROTHER

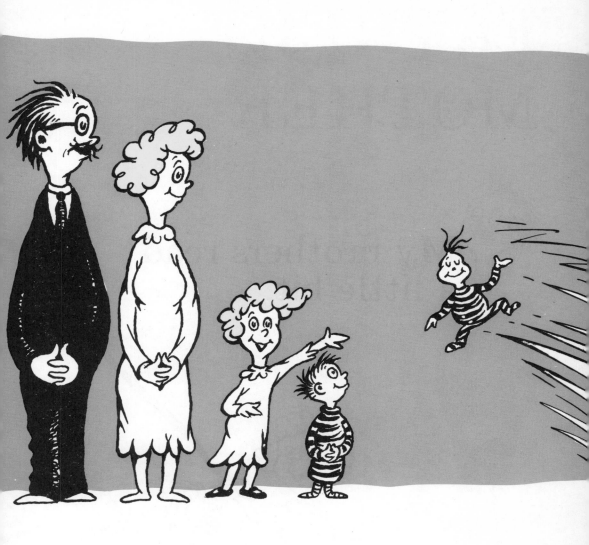

That one is
my other brother.

My brothers read
a little bit.

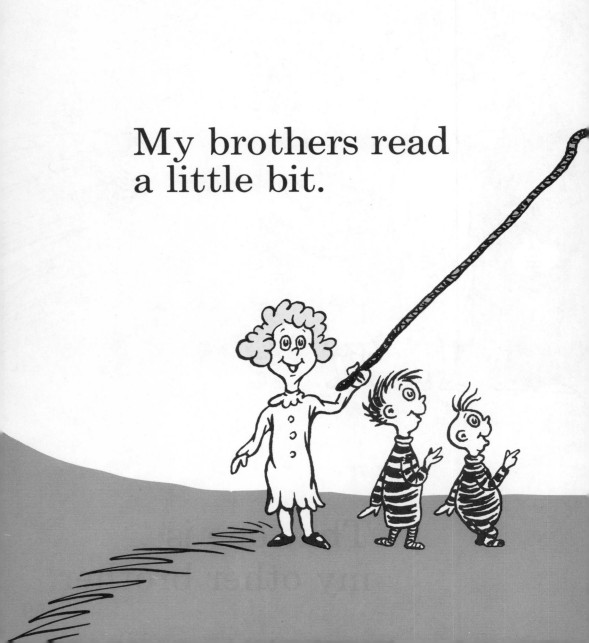

Little
words
like

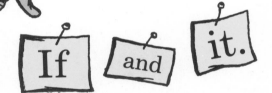

If and it.

My father
can read
big words, too

like......·····

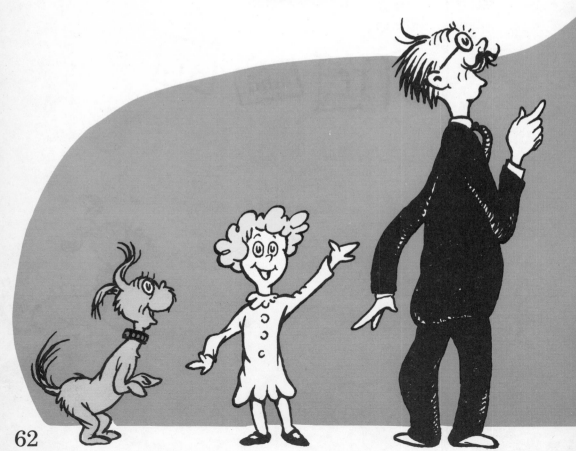

CONSTANTINOPLE

and

TIMBUKTU

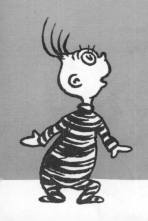
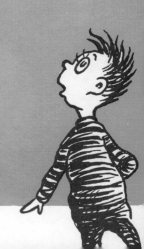

SAY
SAY

What does this say?

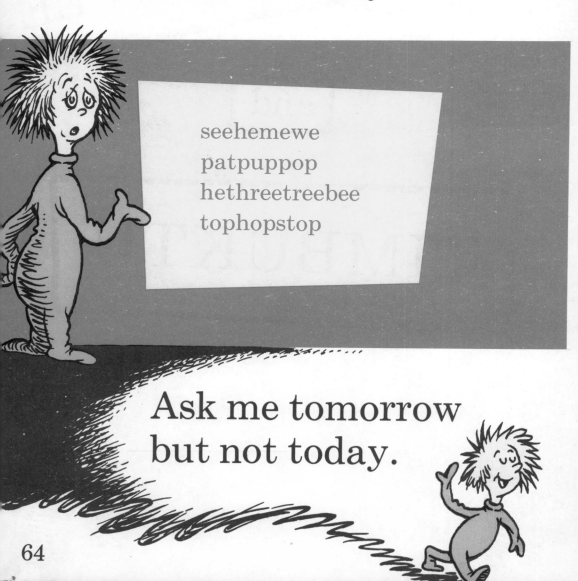

seehemewe
patpuppop
hethreetreebee
tophopstop

Ask me tomorrow
but not today.